T0147637

MILLER'S DIET TIME
IS HERE
FOR WEIGHT LOSS & HEALTH

MILLER'S DIET TIME
IS HERE
FOR WEIGHT LOSS & HEALTH

There is a stimulus package for better health and weight!

R.D. Miller, M.D.

iUniverse, Inc.
New York Bloomington

iUniverse books may be ordered through booksellers or by contacting:

*iUniverse
1663 Liberty Drive
Bloomington, IN 47403
www.iuniverse.com
1-800-Authors (1-800-288-4677)*

*Because of the dynamic nature of the Internet, any Web addresses or
links contained in this book may have changed since publication and
may no longer be valid. The views expressed in this work are solely those
of the author and do not necessarily reflect the views of the publisher,
and the publisher hereby disclaims any responsibility for them.*

*ISBN: 978-1-4401-6462-0 (sc)
ISBN: 978-1-4401-6463-7 (ebook)*

Printed in the United States of America

iUniverse rev. date:08/20/09

Table of Contents

When our creator made the body it had within it what was needed to be healthy and at ideal weight. All we have to do is give it the right things in the right amounts of each when eating and let it happen.

Do you know the name of the country that has everything in place to be the healthiest, trimmest country in the world?

The answer is on page 61

INSIDE THIS
BOOK
IS YOUR
KEY OF
KNOWLEDGE.

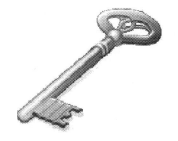

After seeing thousands of patients which convinced me that people need a weight loss book, that is easy to read, understand and apply. It would have to work at home, while traveling, on vacations, when eating fast food in all kinds of restaurants and Mom's home cooking. This is the book that can change your life and your future.

Confusion, frustration and not knowing what the problem is with weight and then keeping it off can be in your past as it should be, and is for myself and many others. In this book you learn and practice a few simple things at every meal. The magnitude is so big it's astounding.

Any change in your eating or health care management should be with approval of your primary care physician, internist, specialist or doctor treating you for a special problem. This is necessary before beginning any weight loss program. Much of the important information is from the academic arena, journals, seminars, research and clinical practice scenarios.

I know what it is to struggle with weight loss trying everything, but I was fortunate enough to meet one of the smartest doctors I have ever known who explained it all to me and I have not had a weight problem since. You will be joining me as you see for yourself.

Being Accepted

Throughout life everyone should experience the feeling that comes with being accepted. Maybe it comes in the form of a phone call that you are being invited into your favorite fraternity or sorority. Or it could be something as life changing as a promotion in your workplace that demonstrates the confidence and belief that your company has in you.

People with a severe weight problem know the disappointment of being passed over for a position they are qualified for or shunned at a social event. This is wrong but everyone with a weight problem knows it happens.

Recently I consoled a patient named Cora, while crying she explained how upset she was because her husband told her she was getting fat! Why would Cora's husband say something so negative to make her feel so rejected? We can't change other people or the way they act, we can only change ourselves.

In the dormitory where I roomed in college I met a blind student that wanted to be friends and didn't know how to go about it. One day I took his cane out of his hand and told him, "You look strong and we're going to wrestle until one of us says that's enough you win!" He agreed so we wrestled until we were hitting the walls, falling on the floor lasting about three to five minutes, until he won the fight fair and square. It wasn't long before several other guys wanted to take him on as well, only then did he feel he was one of us finally accepted.

At our graduation I went up to my friend and said, "I'm going to miss you, even though I never beat you at wrestling." I could see a tear slowly falling down his face, what he couldn't see was the tear coming down my face as well.

Losing weight can be hard or easy depending on whether a person understands the simple basics explained in this book.

Modern Day Moses

In 1987 Dr. Gerald Reaven (our modern day Moses) Professor of Medicine at Stanford University enlightened the medical world with his paper on Syndrome X showing that "The life of the FLESH is in the blood."

By keeping blood sugar and insulin in the normal range cholesterol components are improved, less abdominal obesity, hypertension, diabetes, heart attacks and strokes. Our life is in the blood by carrying oxygen and nutrients to every cell.

Many centuries ago another man well learned in the wisdom of the Egyptians, wrote the same thing Dr. Reaven wrote.

It was Moses who wrote the book of Leviticus in the Bible. Leviticus 17:11 "For the life of the flesh is in the blood."

Forward

How do you become more energized in your daily life? This question has plagued the thoughts of many living in the constantly changing, fast-paced, fast food world. Gaining the energy to make it through your daily life is as simple as reviewing your lifestyle and eating habits. Changing these two aspects of your life will allow moderate weight loss each month and a longer healthier life. In regards to your looks and self-esteem, all that you hoped and longed for can be achieved through these few but necessary alterations.

Most people fail to understand the simplicity involved in gaining energy and losing weight because of a lack of knowledge.

Many are unaware of some simple body chemistries taking place when certain foods are eaten. Some of these foods surprisingly can help you lose weight although you might believe them to cause you to gain weight.

As a weight loss physician, I understand and also relate to you as a reader struggling with weight loss. Years ago, I struggled with a weight problem which no longer hinders my daily life because I have learned new concepts and applied them to my everyday lifestyle so that struggle is now considered part of my past.

Everything I learned through my transformation is offered to you through this book, and these simple changes can be made no matter what type of lifestyle you live.

In college my English professor who was a very nice lady gave me a C (I should have got a D) and she said, "We know you are good in chemistry and glad you're going to be a doctor and not in English.

A Good Example

You may be the only weight loss book someone will ever read.

People with a weight problem are constantly hoping to find that easy diet that works, from Mom's home cooking to fast food or gourmet specialty meals. In reality the plan has to work wherever you dine.

An exciting and happy day is when you join me and others who never think of food or weight because your eating habits have become a natural part of your daily life.

Insurance companies could save billions of dollars on health care costs if they rewarded people who lost weight instead of paying out for medical care, prescriptions, and hospitalization due to being an obese society. This could be done by reducing premiums while awarding a yearly bonus instead of yearly increase to the ever rising medical and insurance costs. The lack of understanding is costing the insurance industry and the overweight patient a fortune. The real loss is the life of the overweight patient.

REWARD THE LOSER!

This would make a good bumper sticker.

The Obesity Epidemic

Are you aware that nearly 400,000 people lose their lives each year attributed to obesity and over ninety billion dollars is spent for their health care costs?

Just about everyone who can be overweight is. Our country has been the leader in almost everything. Being a medical doctor I'm ashamed to admit we are the leader in the obesity epidemic which is becoming a worldwide epidemic.

For more than thirty years most of us were led to believe that low fat - high carbohydrate diets were the healthiest diets recommended, nothing could be further from the truth.

Do you have low energy? After working all day you finally get home, flop down in the big over stuffed chair, click the TV on, grab a cold drink and a bag of chips then wonder if there is something sweet around like chocolate cake not realizing what just happened.

The cravings you just experienced comes from spiking blood sugar levels which is the direct result of eating white bread, cookies, crackers, chocolate, doughnuts, or whatever carbohydrate or sugar you recently consumed. A better choice would be to eat mixed nuts, assorted vegetables or even a piece of fruit.

The major changes concerning our health are high blood pressure, diabetes, and high triglyceride levels. These are related to the high carbohydrate consumption with adults and children. We are now seeing blood pressure elevations and insulin resistance developing in children. Insulin resistance is when blood cells are flooded with too much sugar making insulin have a harder time getting into cells, which makes the pancreas over worked, soon wearing out producing full blown diabetes.

The remedy is what I tell all my patients over and over until it sinks in. We need to keep blood sugar and insulin in the normal range as much as possible, because it's the fat making part of the hormones from the pancreas. The other is glucagon which works with your insulin, not alone. This part is the fat mobilizer that is stimulated by protein and also helps weight loss.

We need to increase our proteins to at least fifty grams per day. I consume at least eighty grams a day which as you see by the example below is very simple to follow.

Example:

•	1 Chicken Breast	30 grams
•	1 Bowl of Special K Protein Cereal	10 grams
•	2 Eggs with 1 Sausage Patty	17 grams
•	1 Small Bowl Tuna Salad w/ 2-crackers	25 grams
	Total	82 grams

Join the club of the few people who are in control of their weight while having less of the side effects that obesity causes by knowing the protein content of the food you eat. You will enjoy having control of what you are eating especially when you see the weight coming down by having the knowledge of what you are doing instead of going through life guessing.

*See protein content food sheet on page 50.

"Self delusion is pulling in your stomach when you step on the scales."

Urgency

Some patients think I come across too strong when talking about the consequences of obesity when they came to my office to lose that weight for the wedding, class reunion or trip to the beach. They do not want to hear a lecture most don't want to hear about heart attacks, strokes, diabetes or high blood pressure problems either, thinking it applies only to others, treating it lightly not realizing the seriousness which could take their life.

I had reservations about writing this chapter and you'll know why when you read this. However it's not right to you if I don't share with you the reason for urgency and seriousness which I hope you will understand.

Years ago I contacted John, a close friend from medical school who was overweight. While visiting his beautiful home I talked to him about losing weight and how I was concerned about his health.

He gave me the courtesy to go over the how and why of a good weight loss program. Finally he said, "All that doesn't apply to me, I lift weights and I don't want to hear anymore." "Ok, you know I'm your friend, I'll not mention it again. Let's go out to the back yard, I want to see that beautiful garden and pool." As I was leaving we agreed to go to Florida together the next summer for our family vacations.

Six months later my wife told me my dear friend John died. That was 18 years ago. His wife sold their home and is now living in another state. You see, I didn't just happen to be in the neighborhood when I met John at his home years ago. I went out of concern for his health. That day I tried to help him, and he rejected my help. Now my dear friend is gone, no longer around for his family. I still grieve the loss of my dear friend John.

You're thinking well that's just one case like that. No not at all, about a year later I spent the afternoon with my study partner from school who was also courteous to me while I tried to share my concern with him about his weight problem. What I received was no interest and a similar story. He had a stroke and went into a coma for a month before he died. This was seventeen years ago. There were other physician friends of mine who were not interested in what I had to say about weight loss that have been gone now for about ten to twelve years.

Just because a person is a doctor doesn't mean he's exempt. Obesity related diseases do not discriminate based on occupation, gender, race, social economic standing or your belief that it will not happen to you. There are always going to be some people that no matter how much you have the desire to help them, they are just not willing to change their eating habits for whatever reason they do not relate the problem to themselves.

What are Free Radicals?

If you knew of something that would slow down aging, give you a better chance to live longer healthier and a minimum of disability you would want to know about it wouldn't you? We all would like to have less of the age related diseases like high blood pressure or cancer and learning about oxidation will help tremendously.

We and other living matter including plants must have oxygen to live and is our metabolic fire that burns within us producing life for us all. We would never think of oxygen as being harmful or being necessary for life, but when oxygen is burned creating energy there are waste products which are water and oxygen based free radicals which are now reactive cells. Fortunately for us these are neutralized instantly but some do escape. Look at it like this, when our car burns gasoline and oxygen it gives the energy that drives it and also has waste products which are water and carbon dioxide.

In our modern world we are assaulted with other harmful things that increase free radicals which are abnormal cells that were once normal and were changed in the oxidation process (burning oxygen). Other things that increase these abnormal cells known as free radicals are cigarette smoke, smog or air pollution, industrial toxins, chemicals in food and water, drugs or medicines, and radiation. When we cut an apple and it immediately starts turning brown that is oxidation and an old car turning to rust is also oxidation.

It's oxidation that ages our tissue in our body causing skin to wrinkle, joint arthritic changes, cataracts, and damaging cells promoting development of cancer.

Another example is when free radicals attach the bad cholesterol which is the LDL or low density lipoprotein, the cholesterol is more sticky and attaches to rough spots on the artery walls and plaques are formed then clogging up causing heart attacks.

Free radicals are also produced more when there is sickness and the longer the illness the more radicals are formed.

What can we do about all this? Avoid as many things mentioned such as smoke and other pollutions. Eating healthier with your new lifestyle and eating more fruits and vegetables and taking antioxidant supplements like Vitamin C, E and Selenium. It's imperative that we keep our immune systems in top performance because cells here track down and find free radicals, destroy them and get rid of many.

I take everything mentioned at the end of the book on vitamins.

In summing all this up, we have billions of cells in our body and about the same amount of atoms. There are about the same number positive charged ones as negative and as long as there about equal we're ok, it's when the balance is interrupted or uncontrolled then the problem begins. Pollution, smog and smoking and other things mentioned upsets the balance and too many free radicals come into the picture.

In closing researchers in Japan where cigarette use per capita is among the highest in the world but the incidence of lung cancer is among the lowest. They contribute this to eating more fruits and raw vegetables and recommend seven half cups of fruits and vegetables every day.

"Honey, would you start keeping a bowl of fruit on the island in the kitchen and a veggie medley (raw) with dip in the fridge?"

Toxic Load Express

No one is sure as to what causes cancer to appear in the stomach, lungs or colon. So now let's focus on what we do know. Chronic irritation from smoking causes cell linings of the bronchial tubes and lungs to change from normal to abnormal, which then becomes cancerous.

Most people know about chronic irritation from allergies with sinusitis, red itchy eyes, runny nose and irritable bowel brought on by some foods.

Some chemicals used in growing food, chlorine, water pollution, nitrates in meat, food additives with coloring, bacteria, viruses, and medicines which have not been absorbed remain in the bowel for long periods of time with irritating effects. This has become known as the toxic load.

Let's consider an interesting thought about a section of Africa where no chlorine was found and preservatives were not present in food. As a result less toxins were found in the bowel and cancer of the colon was extremely rare.

I am not saying that the things in the bowel which are irritating cause cancer, but only time and research will answer this as we look further into this and new areas.

We need to do everything we can to reduce the concentration of these harmful and possible cancer causing toxins, and do all we can to move everything through the bowel faster and regularly. Increasing water intake and fresh fruit and vegetables eaten 6 to 8 times a day will help tremendously. I have seen excellent results with fish oil capsules, one after each meal, 2 or 3 times a day (1,000 mg each). This will also improve the immune system which will help your heart and lessen joint problems.

When I have a patient who has a problem being regular with bowel movements and sometimes need laxatives or a fleet enema my recommendation is to first try fish oil capsules, which

I use regularly. Anything we do to get rid of the toxic load is a plus!

Karen

A woman named Karen was seen in my office months ago who was very depressed because her Mother, Alice whom she loves dearly now suffers with Alzheimer's disease. At the time she was in a nursing home and didn't recognize Karen when she went to visit. I shared with Karen to see that she gets 3 of the 1000 mg of fish oil capsules daily, someway, possibly by putting it in her food. Three months later my patient returned and said, "Oh thank you so much my Mother recognizes me now and talks about things we did together. She is also feeding herself, going to the bathroom and she rearranged the furniture in the waiting room."

I have always felt that a treatment that helps a problem could also help prevent it. This is my personal belief and opinion.

I highly recommend Dr. Barry Sears book, "The Miracle of High Dose fish Oil," you will then start taking fish oil as I do when you read about the successes he is familiar with.

"Brain cells come, brain cells go, fat cells live forever."

Fiber In - Fiber Out

There is no way to pick a more boring subject than fiber. No matter how serious and boring this subject is, why don't we both have fun learning the medical information while you're reading and I'm writing?

It is hard to be happy when you're constipated. Would you agree with that? Let's also agree not to use any ugly four letter words when describing a person who is constipated as full of roughage and not any the other four letter word.

Here is where fiber, which we all eat everyday, having no nutritional value but present in abundance in fruits and vegetables comes to the rescue by moving the intestinal contents faster through the colon relieving our problem. Now our well being has returned with the grimace gone and our smile and happiness back. You will definitely have more energy and we guys can hit the golf ball further because we're smaller in the abdomen and can make a better turn in our golf swing. Sometimes I think I need more fiber when I see my ball going over the hill and into the woods.

Memphis and other cities years ago were beautiful, clean, and safe, less crime, violence, child and spouse abusers and now people are afraid in their own homes or in shopping malls. I think poor leadership is the reason because of their episodes of constipation. A good start for some cities would be to provide them more fiber and would have given them more to do instead of talk, talk, and talk!

This is one item tax payers would not mind paying for and would be glad to deliver. Whether you like this fun example or not, I hope you'll never forget that fiber is an acceptable treatment for chronic constipation.

Did you know fiber can bring more happiness to homes all over America? Many people were not blessed with a great

Mother-in-law like I have, so if your Mother-in-law is not great and seems to be a never ending problem, there is hope! All you have to do is increase her fiber intake with out her knowing.

If you are wondering how much fiber we should have everyday it's at least 30 grams. The average American has less than 10 grams and some studies say 5 grams. (Your mother-in-law may take in less than 5 grams). Be sure and hide this book if you do what I suggest!

Over 50 years ago B.D. (before diets) very little was known about fiber. In the medical schools it was not discussed at all and its merits for better health were not known. Our professor said, "When eating lettuce, just eat the green part and don't bother with the stalk or white part because it has no nutritional value." If that lecture was given today, the professor might say, "When eating lettuce be sure you get plenty of the white section, it may be better for you than the other because of its enormous amount of fiber which we all know is extremely healthy."

Doctor, "I thought this was a diet - energy book, why have we wondered off the subject and are now on fiber?" Ok, do you ever feel tired after too many sweets or regular soft drinks? Rest assured, I go through the same thing and so do many others because blood sugar and insulin has spiked up and energy went down like the Titanic. "Now explain to me how fiber could have helped in this drastic sinking spell?" The answer is in the following list of "The Amazing Fiber Benefits."

The Amazing Fiber Benefits

1. It gives us a full feeling (satiety) and we eat less.

2. A good goal daily is 25-40 grams and can be achieved with more unprocessed fruits and vegetables which have lots of fiber (which is not a food itself) It's the structural support of plants and often lost when processed.

3. 30 grams a day reduces the risk of colorectal cancer. In the American diet the count is less than 10.

4. In sluggish digestion or constipation we benefit by additional fiber which slows down the absorption of glucose and allows a more gradual release of insulin and a faster normal blood sugar and that in itself promotes energy and weight loss.

5. Increasing fiber in the diet is an effective treatment for chronic constipation.

6. Combine with the toxins in the colon and helps move them out of our body faster which we all want to happen.

7. Helps bacteria normally present in the bowel to more normally stabilized.

8. Studies have shown soluble fiber helps in lowering cholesterol levels and the more fiber used the better is the effect.

9. Increase pancreatic secretions and we also have more soluble bile for better digestion.

I know this is a lot of information to digest, I hope it helps.

"See how many people each day you can make smile, laugh or feel better about themselves. You will be amazed how you feel."

R.D. Miller, M.D.

List of Fiber Count

Kidney Beans - 7 grams

Navy Beans - 6 grams

Baked Beans - 8 grams

Lima Beans - 4 grams

Dried Peas cooked - 4.7 grams

Green Beans - 3 grams

Broccoli - 4.5 grams

Brussels Sprouts - 4.6 grams

Fruit, Medium Size - 3.5 grams

Banana, Medium Size - 2.4 grams

Orange, Medium Size - 2.6 grams

Pear with skin, Large - 3 grams

3 Prunes - 3 grams

Strawberries, 1 Cup - 3 grams

Raspberries, 1/2 Cup - 3 grams

All Bran, 1 bowl - 8.5 grams

Raisin Bran, 1 bowl - 4 grams

Special K Protein Plus, 1 bowl - 5 grams

Research scientists and food companies have obtained an enormous amount of knowledge about the contribution of fiber to better health, more energy, less disease and general feeling of well being.

Subsequently many companies are adding more fiber to their products and Americans are checking product contents for higher fiber count.

Cancer

After all the tests and diagnostic procedures are done the one word no one wants to hear is cancer. It's obvious by the number of people who quit smoking that if anyone could do more to prevent smoking they would.

A cancer cell was once a normal cell, but became abnormal through a changing process brought on by losing the regulation of its growth and becoming a cancerous mass invading the surrounding tissue, then spreading to distant areas. During this process the cells DNA is changing as well as genetic change which we see in cancer of the lungs, colon, breast and brain.

The starting process could come from a chemical, virus, smoke, water, air pollution, chronic irritation (smoking), food additives, pesticides, paint, ozone smog and stress which everyone is familiar with.

Have you noticed you're more likely to get sick during stress? That's because cortisol from the adrenal is produced slowing our immune system down which is our defense mechanism.

Our immune system prevents infections from bacteria, viruses, fungi, and cancer by producing immune cells, T-lymphocytes and anti-tumor chemicals known as interferon. These constantly circulate through the body finding, destroying and removing abnormal cells, defective cells and damaged cells before they multiply, divide and become cancer. This defense system should also be referred to as our prevention system.

Are you aware that some families have a higher risk of developing certain cancers such as breast, ovary, colon and skin?

Another factor increasing cancer risk is cigarette smoke.

In 1930 there were about 5 patients in 100,000 with lung cancer, in 1990 about 110 patients out of 100,000 with lung cancer. In women lung cancer has sky rocketed. In summary there is no one thing we can do or take to keep from getting cancer, but we should do all we know to strengthen our immune system. Things listed below are what I believe in doing and have done for many years. I would like to share with you how I live and what I take daily. Consult with your doctor before starting this regimen.

Elevated blood sugar and insulin depresses the immune system. This is taken care of with proper eating.

Avoid stress as much as possible. Stop using tobacco and use water and air filters when possible.

- Vitamin C - 2000 mg Daily
- Vitamin E - 800 units daily
- B - Complex - 1 daily
- Calcium - 1200 mg Daily
- Magnesium - 400 mg Daily
- Garlic - 2000 mg Daily
- Coenzyme Q-10 - 200 mg Daily
- Selenium - 200 mcg daily
- Ginkgo Biloba - 120 mg Daily
- Fish Oil - 3000 mg Daily

*See chapter on vitamins for more details.

Had A Brazil Nut Lately?

Brazil nuts are loaded with selenium and eating two a day will provide what you need. Selenium is also in whole grains, clams, oysters and lobster. This little powerful trace mineral is a strong antioxidant as shown by many studies and research.

Years ago in China was having more cancer than any other area in China. The government checked the soil and found it to be low in selenium. They then supplied selenium for the people, and the problem was resolved. This started studies and case reports all over the world with astounding findings and information. "Doctor, I'm taking a multivitamin am I going to have to take another pill?" No, but let's make that decision after you see what it does.

This little mysterious trace mineral has received attention for its possible role in cancer prevention and not to replace chemo or treatments being given, but could be a helpful addition.

In 1996 the Journal of the American Medical Association it was reported that selenium given at three times the recommended daily dose gave over 50% fewer cases of prostate cancer, rectal cancer, lung cancer and 50% reduction in total cancer deaths. More studies have since followed these studies.

Most everybody would like to stay as young as they can as long as they can and in the meantime slow down the aging process. It also activates substances that help prevent cataracts, prevents heart muscle damage, boost elements that fights infection, and improves your immune system.

Vitamin E and selenium work together to help neutralize the cell damage done by free radicals which are abnormal oxygen molecules that was once normal.

This is interesting because a cancer cell was at one time a normal cell that became abnormal from whatever cause. Selenium is justly classified as an antioxidant and has been referred to as being a chemo-preventive agent. In many different parts of the world people who have low blood levels of selenium tend to have more cancer in many different organs.

Studies have also shown that selenium improves energy, better mood and less anxiousness or depression. I believe in it and I currently take 200 micrograms daily.

Have you decided yet to take another pill?

Do you know how Freddy Mack and Fannie Mae caused weight gain? People made a bee line to the comfort foods, tranquilizers, and over to the couch and said, "To heck with it all especially the exercise!"

The Maidenhair Tree

Years ago when my daughter was three we had a tree next to our home and in the fall when all the leaves fell which took about a week, the ground was the brightest yellow you ever saw. I put a small stool in the middle of them and had my daughter sit there with a red dress on and the beauty of that picture was unbelievable. Of course the little girl who was my daughter had nothing to do with it being a beautiful picture. I didn't realize at the time that I was walking on those leaves and hidden there was a fantastic medicine that would improve concentration, memory, energy, depression, dizziness and tinnitus which is ringing of the ear. Also, it's showing improvement in dementia and Alzheimer's.

There's a beautiful tree that grows in China called the Maidenhair Tree. In the fall when all the leaves fall, the ground is covered with beautiful bright yellow leaves making an excellent spot for picture taking.

The Maidenhair Tree of China is known in this country as the ginkgo tree which many are familiar with. A medicine has been found in the beautiful yellow leaves which have some surprising benefits. It has an affect on your memory which will astound you as you remember names and events of many years ago. It also improves your learning and thinking ability. I can personally testify to this and when you experience it you'll understand. It is presumed to help by increasing oxygen flow to the brain protecting it from free radical damage, and may curb the symptoms of Alzheimer's disease.

I believe the cure for cancer is hidden in a tree leaf that hasn't been discovered. Now consider medicines from leaves we have found. Witch doctors years ago made a mixture in a big black pot, said some voodoo chants and gave it to people who did recover from some illnesses because of the digitalis leaf.

We use it today for heart conditions. Long ago certain countries sent large sail boats to other countries to get boat loads of aloe leaves which are on the shelves of every store as mixtures for healthy skin. Then there were peppermint leaves for digestion and bowel spasms relieved with a medicine from the belladonna leaf.

Mary

Months ago a friend of mine, Mary told me about her Mother, Hilda who was suffering with Alzheimer's and currently resides in a nursing home. Hilda did not recognize her daughter Mary during visits, and while Hilda was bedridden and fought to be fed, Mary worried about her Mother. One day Mary asked me if I knew of anything that would help her Mother. I told her I could not guarantee anything but if Hilda were my Mother I would make sure she got two ginkgo biloba with her food daily. Mary did this and in less than three months her Mother recognized her, talked, fed herself and sits some in the waiting room. She was very grateful for the change in her Mother.

Studies from Columbia University in New York have shown that vitamin E may also slow progression of Alzheimer's. Treatment of this nature should be approved by the physician treating the patient.

Some other things ginkgo has been thought to do are improve mood, circulation, decreasing blood clotting, more oxygen to different parts of the body helping blood vessel damage to the eye from diabetes and improves circulation to the legs which could relieve cramping.

A patient of mine named Joann, told me she had a ringing in her right ear that was driving her crazy. We have a lot of good ear doctors in the Memphis area so I referred her to one for treatment.

After two months and no results, I said, "Do something for a trial, take 120 mg of ginkgo daily as I do, which will cost around $10.00." She did and in two days the ringing in her ears stopped.

This little pill is fabulous. I take 120 mg daily and will from now on!

"In the midst of the street of and on either side of the river, was there the tree of life, which bare twelve manners of fruits, and yielded her fruit every month; and the leaves of the tree were for the healing of the nations." Revelations 22:2

Has God hidden the cure for cancer in a leaf?

Miracle Pill Coenzyme

Are you one of many who feel tired most of the time even though you have had enough rest? I could not count the times when seeing a new patient they say, "Be sure to check my thyroid, which may be low as the problem runs in my family." Others ask if vitamins, sleeping pills or something for stress or depression will help. They are looking for a reason that they don't feel at all like they used to.

We in the medical world have not even touched the surface when it comes to understanding the function of all our organs, hormones and the immune system which protects us from many diseases and infections. Then consider the blood which carries oxygen and nutrients to cells and while making the delivery picks up the waste and carries it away for removal. With all this and the heart pumping constantly it's good to know that each one of our cells has an energy factory called mitochondria which does the job but needs a spark to begin work at full capacity producing energy we need with many other health benefits.

This amazing vitamin like substance known as Coenzyme Q-10 which is the spark manufactured in our body from the amino acid tyrosine with the aid of Vitamin B - 12, Vitamin B - 6, Niacin and Vitamin C, and when these are deficient as in a poor diet we make less coenzymes. Also it is fat soluble and needs to be taken with a fatty meat or small amount of peanut butter.

Some of the first studies were done in Japan in the 1950's that believed energy was its only function. By 1960 many physicians were noticing great improvement in their congestive heart failure patients, other cardiac problems and twice as much coenzyme was found in the heart than other organs. By 1980 it was one of the top five selling drugs and many more studies have since been done in our country.

More and more nutrition oriented doctors are learning about this little known vitamin like nutrient essential in the body's production of energy, and now on the horizon looking as an aide to help in many heart problems, not as a replacement, but in conjunction with what is being used.

Carl

A few years later my mechanic friend Carl was taken to the hospital with a heart attack and lived one year. His wife told me the doctor said he had cardiomyopthy and nothing could be done. I will always wonder about what might have happened if coenzyme had been given to Carl.

Coenzyme is normally concentrated in the heart muscle and less amount present when weakened with age, many years of high blood pressure, heart attacks, diabetes or alcohol abuse or the body not making as much as we need.

It's also been shown to lower cholesterol by combining with the bad one (LDL) and more coenzyme present the better the effect, also necessary for the optimal functioning of the immune system.

Studies have shown that breast cancer patients have a coenzyme deficiency and it's reasonable to me that it could also aid in prevention. Dr. Karl Folkers at the University of Texas has done extensive research with coenzyme and reported remissions with metastatic breast cancer and Dr. Lockwood and colleagues report favorable results and should be given in conjunction with conventional therapy.

The Coenzyme Q-10 researcher Dr. Peter Langsjoen a Cardiologist in Tyler, Texas says, in some people improvement is clear and many times dramatic. In cardiomyopthy the heart muscle slowly stops functioning becoming weaker and coenzyme helps the remaining muscle do the job better.

Ted

Twenty years ago a very close friend told me his daughter had developed cardiomyopthy after her pregnancy. She was extremely anxious and worried after being informed that this could take her life. He asked me if I knew anything that might be done. I told him if she was my daughter, I would start her on Coenzyme today, three to four hundred milligrams daily and I wasn't sure it would help, but would do no harm.

He started her on it that day. It was amazing in three to four weeks she was doing some things around the house and slowly started caring for the baby. Improvement was seen every day and three months later she was doing everything as before with complete recovery.

At this point you're thinking with all the studies, "Why haven't we not heard of this before?" I thought the same thing as my father and my wife's father died with congestive heart failure and no mention of coenzyme was made. I think the reason is you can buy it over the counter in the vitamin section in super stores being a natural product. It would cost pharmaceutical companies a great deal of money just for a patent and would not be feasible to manufacture or distribute.

With more studies and time I'm sure we will all be more aware of the miracle pill which I still take 200 mg daily.

Cholesterol

When we think of the complexity of cholesterol, it reminds me of the Ladies, not all good and not all bad, but a little of each and sometimes more of one than the other.

It's waxy in substance, not soluble in water, and not dissolving in blood which has a very high percentage of water, so our body coats it with protein to allow transportation through our blood stream. This is where the term lipoprotein comes from and has two parts, the healthy one picks up cholesterol from cells and take it to the liver, this one is referred to as HDL or healthy one. The other brings cholesterol to cells and is known as LDL and it is not healthy.

Cholesterol is definitely essential to life, we can't live without it and most is in every cell doing good, like regulating nutrients going in and out, helping strengthen the wall while disposing of waste. It's the starting point for making important hormones: The sex hormones testosterone and estrogen, adrenal hormones helping regulate blood pressure and makes hydrocortisone, repairs tissue, a big component in bile acids, and for healthy brain and nervous tissue.

Let's look at triglycerides which I think is more important than just looking at the total cholesterol. Blood sugar and insulin level rises up from eating too much of the foods we have talked about is what makes triglycerides elevated. The reason it is dangerous is because it makes your blood thicker, sludgy and clots blocking arteries.

I recently saw a patient when we drew his blood, one half of the test tube (bottom part was red, but the upper half looked like buttermilk), his triglycerides were 1,080 (normal is below 100).

He was extremely obese and ate too much of the wrong things all the time. In my mind he was a heart attack walking around. He is now losing weight the right way and the cholesterol and triglycerides will be normal in a few months because he listened to me (I scared him good!)

The first test I look for is the triglycerides, HDL ratio which is for

Example:

1 triglyceride/1 HDL - Good

2 triglyceride/1 HDL - Borderline Normal

Very rarely I see a patient with the HDL higher than the triglycerides such s triglycerides 75/HDL - 100 - this is great!

If you have your lab sheet you can check your ratio. Follow the eating plan in this book and your levels will straighten out.

Russian Penicillin

Centuries ago in Europe when one army defeated another army and took over, one of the first things they did was to plant garlic around the walls. They thought of garlic as a cure and tonic for infections of all kinds, bowel problems, and unhealthy blood. We have since learned of the many health benefits of garlic. Garlic kills seventy two different bacteria, viruses, fungi; it thins the blood and acts as an anti-inflammatory agent. I sometimes wonder what else the medical people in those armies, centuries ago, knew that was not written down, such as putting it on infected wounds or making a liquid broth.

I want to share with you how what we've learned can help us in our daily lives whether at home or traveling in foreign countries. I visited the Holy Lands in 1970 which was thirty five years ago B.T. (before terrorism). Traveling through Athens and Greece I visited the Parthenon remains with large columns, stones and unbelievable workmanship. I went up the mountain alone as everyone on the bus was sick (probably caused by something in the food eaten at a previous restaurant where we ate), I was glad I took three Russian penicillin pills that day (garlic) instead of two as usual.

Peter

I shared this with a friend, Peter who had business in India every two months and was sick most of the time while there. He was losing ten to fifteen pounds from diarrhea and poor appetite. On his next trip he took one garlic pill after each meal, and one at bedtime. After returning he told me how great the trip was, no sickness or diarrhea and was very grateful for telling him about taking the garlic pills. He was looking forward to his next trip. I take three or four garlic pills daily when traveling to foreign countries.

I was once asked if I knew anything that can be done or used on lip and mouth sores that are very irritating and painful. Many times this is the herpes simplex virus which will respond after taking two garlic capsules a day and taken indefinitely.

He did this with no recurrence in ten years. A similar thing was accomplished with a person who had genital herpes for several years and no matter what was done or taken the problem continued, he also took garlic two times a day with no recurrence in over five years. These types of cases never cease to astound me! No wonder someone named garlic the Russian penicillin.

Many times I have patients say to me, "I have seen the ad's on TV for different meds for cholesterol, which one do you recommend?" When I first see a patient with elevated cholesterol I tell them what I take and have for many years keeping it in the normal range at 160.

I take B - Complex and two garlic tablets each day after eating. About fifty percent of cholesterol is made in the liver and garlic blocks its production, and the B mixture helps the liver function better aiding the blockage. I tell my patients to try this before beginning meds and if already on medicine then continue on as I never interfere with other doctor's treatments. Consider this, 50% of cholesterol is made in the liver and we block its production, doesn't it make common sense that our cholesterol would probably be in the normal range or become less? We hear about good cholesterol and bad cholesterol, garlic straightens them out.

I also believe elevated or spiking blood sugar with elevated insulin stimulates the liver to make more cholesterol and the new lifestyle concerning your eating learned in this book will take care of this. You will be pleased to see what these three will do for your cholesterol, (Garlic, B - Complex and eating right). This reminds me of Archie Peyton and Eli Manning.

Garlic will also help you to handle stress and depression better by triggering the release of serotonin which is the precursor in forming Prozac which we all know is an anti-depressant.

Garlic can lower blood pressure and prevent heart attacks by thinning the blood with less sticking together of the platelets and decreasing leg pain by increasing the blood flow.

On the first page of a textbook in Urology was written: Garlic and onion help clean your arteries. I have always wondered why that was placed in a book on Urology.

It's Not Good To Rush

Sometimes it's not a good thing to lose too much weight too fast. A gradual consistent weight loss is much better for you.

A friend of mine needed to lose about 50 pounds because of high blood pressure. He farmed 10,000 acres which he had acquired through hard work and good business sense. Now with excellent help on his farm he became more sedate and before he knew it he was over weight. Eating fast food and not exercising was taking its toll on him.

The following month, after sticking with this plan he was excited and telling everyone in the office how great he felt by losing twenty six pounds in his first month. His first words to me were, "I haven't had any bread or potatoes at all, not even a little bite since I started seeing you!"

This is the one thing I hated to hear more than anything, and I knew I would probably never see my friend again. The feeling of being deprived takes over at some point and when people push hard and fast to lose weight they tend to over do it and gain more weight back, which he did. There is no way for me to tell you how many similar cases I have seen like this. Moderation at the beginning is extremely hard to teach because patients want the weight off so bad they are ready to do anything as long as it's fast. We have become an instant gratification society which makes it hard for the patient to be patient.

If I don't explain things like this to you then I'm at fault because you're doing something that will not work. If he had not cut things out completely but cut them back then my friend would have continued to lose weight and he would now have been at his ideal weight, happier, more energetic with normal blood pressure, and enjoying trips and vacations that he deserved after years of hard work.

To sum it up, what a shame to fail when he could have been successful without the rush.

If you must miss some points I make, PLEASE don't miss this one.

I hope you will think like a runner in a marathon starting at a comfortable pace with the intention of finishing the race. Don't be a sprinter running hard and fast to only have the race end right after you started. Have a weekly and monthly goal and reward yourself when one goal is reached.

The following is one of my favorite examples.

Laura

A lady patient named Laura came to my office years ago, each month Laura would lose weight, the first month she lost 2 pounds, the next month she gained 3 pounds, the next month she lost 1 pound, the next month she broke even. Then Laura came in and had lost 7 pounds in one month. She would continue to lose at a rate of 6 to 8 pounds per month for 10 months with 70 pounds total weight loss. I asked Laura to explain to me what happened, she said, "I decided to start listening."

In Between Meals

The reason the right snack is very important mid morning or afternoon is preventing up and down swings in blood sugar which is the culprit creating more hunger, tiredness, mood swings, irritability and changes in focus and energy. Planning your snacks will help alleviate a lot of this suffering. Many people on weight loss programs don't realize how enjoyable or helpful a snack can be.

The wrong snack can create havoc by spiking blood sugar and you think "that was great, what a relief." A little later blood sugar plunges now you're hungrier than before and all those bad feelings return. Many do this several times a day. Now you begin to have all sorts of thoughts wondering if your metabolism is too low or low thyroid like some of your kin. I understand your frustration and awful feeling. You are not alone, overweight people everywhere are experiencing the same thing.

I do not believe a person will ever take control until they master the snack, which is definitely needed and helps when done right.

Here is one example how snacks can decrease hunger:

Years ago in the doctor's dining room many would arrive fifteen or twenty minutes early and have discussions of the events of the day. On the table there were crackers, horseradish and catsup. Many would top a cracker with horseradish and catsup NOT realizing how this would decrease their hunger. Smaller orders were given resulting in much less food distributed and being NOTED by the staff, crackers and other things were removed and orders resumed as before.

Let snacks help you with controlling weight. Protein will help you lose weight with snacks. Include this in your thinking when making choices.

My favorite mid-morning snack.

We know that natural foods in the raw, natural in the whole form, still having the outer shell which is bran, also contains fiber slowing down digestion allowing blood sugar to rise slowly.

Examples:

Whole wheat flour, brown rice, popcorn (Yes, we can have popcorn at the movies!), all whole fruits and all fresh and frozen vegetables. These are known as complex carbohydrates, very healthy and aids in weight loss. The veggie medley with broccoli, cauliflower and carrots is the one I like with a cheese dip and I have most days.

Example:

In a Mexican restaurant for an appetizer or any snack, have guacamole dip which is high in protein. I realize you are thinking, "That's high fat," sure is but monounsaturated fat is very healthy and used in the Mediterranean diet with less heart problems. Just use more dip and less chips! A hard boiled egg with 6 grams of protein, chicken nuggets or a piece of lunch meat from the refrigerator is also good.

Consider a protein bar or shake, assorted vegetables with cauliflower, broccoli and baby carrots, two each with cheese sauce. A piece of fresh fruit, 1/2 apple, 1/2 orange, 4 or 5 grapes, plums, peach, strawberries, half a grapefruit, 3 small celery with dip. Once in awhile have a banana, because a banana is 28 grams of carbohydrate. When I snack I like to eat 15-20 deluxe mixed nuts.

I am often asked if it's OK to eat before going to bed. Why not? Protein helps us lose weight so sometimes I eat a few pieces of turkey and a small glass of milk, both have tryptophane which is the precursor to form serotonin in making something like Prozac, so you will be losing weight and sleeping better than most!

Your pancreas doesn't know whether the moon is out or if the sun is shining, it will respond to what's there, and we still have a few low fat, high carb thinkers, believe it or not.

Girl: *I'd like a triple vanilla sundae with chocolate syrup, nuts, and whipping crème, topped with a slice of cucumber*

Waiter: *Did I hear you right? Did you say top it off with a slice of cucumber?*

Girl: *Good heavens, you're right! Forget the cucumber, I'm on a diet.*

The Fifties

Fifty years ago B.D. (before diets) losing weight and keeping it off was not as difficult as we see today even though we have more books, clinics, trainers, weight loss clinics and doctors in that specialty. In those years it was common knowledge and done by movie stars, dancers, celebrities, models and others who wanted to be trim for whatever reason. "If it was so good why haven't we heard about it?" For some reason it was lost and we're left with the problem everywhere. More and more people entered the weight loss arena bringing new methods and ideas which didn't result in sustained weight loss.

This conglomerated mess created confusion, indecision and mass obesity.

The secrets lost are in this book and will guide you out of your confusion as it has me for many years.

Losing weight is one of the hardest things if you are not familiar with basics and know what you are doing. When you do you'll find it's astoundingly easy.

A new patient should not be over loaded with too much information and should begin to see success while developing confidence. People usually want to lose a lot of weight quickly, but I'm very happy when it's between five and ten pounds the first month. I give a reminder every visit, "I'm doing everything you are, every meal and every snack you are not alone."

Many people are not aware that stress makes you gain weight, because we head for the comfort foods resulting in more cortisone from the adrenal gland and stress related actions.

Stresses come from many sources, a family problem, and loss of work, separation or financial situation.

By being a good listener on my part now comes into play and I can help identify what triggers. In the beginning we need to learn a little of the basic chemistry of food in relation to your body and do a few staple things for the first month, because too much thinking of what to do or wondering if we can eat this or that is not a good idea. Let's focus on three major foods that turn to sugar and creating the fat, which are constantly in front of you, me and everybody else in America every time we eat. Bread, potatoes, and sweets which we all love.

Does it sound reasonable, if we ate less of these each time and not quit completely, we would have less fat being made? That's exactly what happens and continue other things as before. Why don't we say, eat less pasta, corn or pizza? OK, but how many times do we have these for breakfast, probably never, but the three we mentioned are at every meal so we're having less of the problem no matter where we're at from fast food, home, restaurants, traveling, business meetings or wherever we find ourselves each day. It has to be this way, the other will not work.

After going over this and giving some examples like one piece of toast with eggs and bacon, taking the top off a hamburger or sandwich, less of the fries or baked potato and when finished less of the dessert. We are now beginning to develop the habit of eating less bread and potatoes at every meal. We have only two things to think about at meals and confusion is out of the picture. The meals over, now eat less dessert.

Anytime there is not weight loss the problem is usually easy to find and correct.

Also, at each visit a comment is made about increasing protein with an extra piece of chicken, turkey, beef, fish or deviled egg. This stimulates the hormone to help lose weight, change to the diet drink and use less artificial sweeteners.

Have a snack mid morning and afternoon with fruit, mixed nuts, assorted vegetables with the dip you like or a protein bar with low carbohydrates. These are some of the things I do.

People don't realize it, but from day one they are learning how to do maintenance which is the proper habits being formed, which usually take sixty to ninety days and then all becomes natural and weight problems are less and less.

When a patient is not losing and doing as told, then it's our job to find the problem. First culprit with the ladies is usually chocolate and that can't be helped because they do have a chocolate lobe somewhere in the brain, and we have not located the chocolate lobe yet even on CAT scans, but I believe it's there. Don't worry ladies someday it will be found!

To stop the chocolate craze which is rampant everywhere a substitution will have to be developed. I recommend a small apple, orange, five or six olives, tomato juice, mixed nuts, or protein such as chicken nuggets, sugar free Jell-O gelatin, or an assortment of vegetables with cheese sauce or a dip you like.

Too many artificial sweeteners are another common reason people are not losing weight. The sweetness stimulates the taste buds on your tongue and in your mouth. Which sends a message to the pancreas to get the insulin up as a big carbohydrate meal is on the way, but actually it's not.

I saw a man who was putting sweeteners in his coffee all day long. He quit and added a drop of cream in each cup, like I do. When he did this he lost eight pounds. One lady lost five pounds when she replaced sweetener in her tea with lemon. It never ceases to amaze me at the number of people that do this. You see artificial sweetener but your body says sugar. I know you're thinking, "Doc, every time we find something good you take it away, first fried pies and now sweetener." Another thing to consider when weight loss plateaus is exercise which can be done three to four times a week with a fast walk for ten to twenty minutes each time. I go around the block twice, three times a week.

If you think about it five minutes is not long, look at your watch for three minutes and you will see just how long five minutes is. So walk three minutes as fast as you can and just see how you feel. If you are not out of breath and your legs aching then you did not do it fast enough. It's very hard to lose weigh with no exercise and for some people it's impossible. Whatever you do make sure it's fun and enjoyable, then you will want to do it on a regular basis.

"Doctor, earlier you mentioned only three foods to eat less of at each meal, what about all the other foods?" You're right it doesn't sound like much to do at first, but let's look at it a little closer. OK an example is eggs and bacon in the morning, one piece of toast (that's one thing we did by leaving the other piece) at noon don't eat the top of the sandwich (that's 2) in a period of thirty days we have not eaten 60 pieces of bread (the problem) and then eat one-half of the baked potato (15 potatoes not eating in 30 days).

So we do three a day for 7 days which is 21 times a week, multiplied by 4 weeks which equals 84 things a month. I do these things everyday. With no counting. The magnitude of this is astounding.

The only thing on our mind is 2 things at every meal which is bread and potatoes and will eat less each time, then of course less dessert. You ask, "Can I have cheese and macaroni with my meal?" Sure we're not trying to do 85 things we're doing 84.

Doing 84 things is enough for you and me, now you can stop looking around for something else to cut back on and enjoy your meal.

Contrary to what some believe the music of the 50's was not the only great thing of that era. The food rated high on the list and have left great memories for many of us.

Compare the food you ate from your Mother and Grand Mother's kitchen and you'll realize it was easier controlling weight then rather than today in our fast food sandwich pizza world of today. You usually found eggs/meat for breakfast, one or two meats with fresh vegetables for lunch and dinner with very limited dessert and always bread which we eat less of.

When someone loses fifteen pounds or more a large bell in my office is rung. Sometimes a child will ring the bell.

See Yourself There

There are a few very important things which are necessary to have the success you want in losing weight. It is very important to have a vision and a strong dream which will create power to become the person you want to be. Your attitude and belief in yourself will determine if you fulfill your inward desire.

See yourself like you want to be as you take this journey for success. Have weekly, monthly, and a long range goal.

Example:

Losing 2 pounds a week or 10 pounds a month and a final goal while giving yourself a treat small or large each time a goal is met. Some would like a cruise or a week on the beach. See yourself there and keep the vision alive. For some it may be a trip to New York for a new wardrobe. Whatever it is, it will be your dream.

A patient named Pam lost seven pounds the first month, then 9 pounds the second month and 7 pounds the third month. Pam was excited and loving her new found energy level. I asked her what she was doing to be successful on the plan. Pam shared with me that when she shops she looks strictly at protein and anything that says two grams of protein she puts it back and keeps looking until it says fifteen grams then she grabs it. Pam said, "I was skinny and healthy in school and I want to be there again so, when I'm cooking at home my thoughts are on more protein, because it works!"

Exercise

If you are under the care of a physician or specialist for a medical condition you should have their approval before starting any exercise program.

When choosing your exercise program it is absolutely necessary for it to have one ingredient and that is you thoroughly enjoy and look forward to your exercise then you will be successful, and do it for the rest of your life. For example, playing golf a couple of times a week, repetitions with light weights, push-ups, stretching and care of the yard takes care of my exercise and I enjoy each thing.

You may ask, "Do you ride a cart when playing golf?" Yes, I do and I get plenty of walking over hills to find the ball and for some reason my ball is a long way from the cart path. In the winter, all you have to do is put on more clothes and if there has been a light snow then you can play with an orange golf ball which stands out at a distance. Tiger Woods hits his drives 300 plus yards, and one day I beat him with 400 plus yards, the lake was frozen and the ball flew across the ice and ended up on the other side of the lake near the green.

I graduated from high school in 1949 and probably a lot older than you and 20 years older than the guys I play golf with. Nobody has more fun than I do playing golf and I want you to feel the same way about your exercise. I am well aware that what I have just written about my exercise may have been boring, but did you get the impression I love what I do? It is relaxing fun, which you need to find for yourself. Your exercise may be something simple like a brisk walk with a friend, tennis, dancing, hiking, gardening, water or snow skiing, softball, basketball with kids, health clubs with a trainer or using a treadmill while watching TV.

Each person will have to find their niche and when found it will not be like exercise but fun, and do it for the rest of your life and never think of quitting.

Protein is the Secret

What this country has done and is doing now for the last thirty years concerning weight loss and health is obviously wrong. The low fat high carbohydrate plan is the biggest failure ever given to large numbers of people which most have given up. To prove this, sit in a mall and count ten people walking by and see for yourself the number of people you think would be at their ideal weight. You will be shocked and sad to see so many people extremely uncomfortable, in a daze, and have no idea what to do to get their weight down.

I don't believe it would be possible to find a doctor to speak at a medical convention on the merits of low fat high carbohydrate eating. The residual damage is still around because even now patients tell me of a new food their trying and quickly say, "Its low fat." With the low fat, high carbohydrate eating diabetics have a terrible time regulating blood sugar and go from one medicine to another with never ending frustration.

Chrissie

I met a lady named Chrissie who needed to lose 40-50 pounds. On her first visit her blood pressure was 200/120. Chrissie was told to see her local medical doctor or internist today and start on blood pressure medicine as soon as possible. Because of her elevated blood pressure she could have a stroke.

Chrissie was instructed the same as with all new patients. We have two hormones in our body that will help weight come down and we need both working at the same time. When blood sugar and insulin are elevated we put on weight and there are three foods in this country which most people eat too much of, which are bread, potatoes and sweets, that will cause blood sugar elevation.

R.D. Miller, M.D.

Insulin the first hormone to be discussed which we need to bring down to the normal range, is done by eating less of the bread, potatoes and sweets at every meal, which makes many patients lose about 5 pounds a month. If we could get the other hormone in the pancreas up which is made in the alpha cells and known as glucagon we can lose another 4 or 5 pounds. To see glucagon up and insulin down is the key. Glucagon is stimulated by protein so we eat more chicken, turkey, roast, fish, deviled eggs, protein bars, shakes, and some patients add protein powder to oatmeal.

Example:
At Thanksgiving Dinner we have an extra piece of turkey, fish, roast, and deviled egg, half of the roll and a tablespoon of mashed potatoes. It never ceases to amaze me how easy it is to lose weight.

Again Chrissie was told that blood pressure meds were needed and to get that appointment. The next visit she had lost 10 pounds, was eating as instructed, no meds yet, and blood pressure was improving to 180/110. It continued to fall to 160/90 where she is now after losing 35 pounds.

This case is presented to show results from proper eating, correcting blood pressure and weight management. Blood sugar was brought in the normal range along with the master hormone insulin. This hormone affects every cell in the body and you could write a book on its importance. It not only regulates blood sugar as any diabetic knows, but controls the storage of fat. It also regulates making cholesterol and is involved in appetite control.

Consistent elevated blood sugar from eating too much of the high glycemic carbohydrates over many years we see obesity which is obvious around the waist, at the same time developing much more serious silent changes happening in your body.

These silent changes will increase the risk of developing diabetes, cardiovascular disease, abnormal cholesterol, increased fibrinogen level contributing to clot formation. We sure don't want that when thinner blood is better. Cases have also been directed to polycystic ovary disease. You might know of someone who can relate to this. Our answer to help preventing this is protein; our best defense is to increase protein daily to at least 50 grams a day. I'm usually at 75. It's really easy to do when you look about the protein content of foods. Some will surprise you. I believe protein increase is what most need including me.

Summing It Up

Too many carbohydrates and consistent high insulin needs to be decreased and the other hormone glucagon which mobilizes fat for removal needs to be increased. Protein is the stimulus.

We simply reverse what most people do when they are getting more carbohydrates and less protein, now we are getting more protein and less carbohydrates. When you weigh each week you'll be glad as well at seeing your cholesterol going down while at the same time you'll be having less sweet cravings. It never ceases to amaze me how simple this really is and it works anywhere anytime.

FOOD	SERVING SIZE	PROTEIN CONTENT
DAILY VALUE	PROTEIN (DV) =	50-80 GRAMS
Beans, refried	1 Cup	16g
Beef round roast	3 oz.	25g
Black-eyed peas, boiled	1 Cup	13g
Bread	1 Slice	3g
Broccoli	1/2 Cup	3g
Cheddar cheese	2 oz.	14g
Chicken, white meat	3.5 oz.	31g
Chickpeas, boiled	1 Cup	15g
Egg white	1	3g
Egg whole	1`	6g
Feta cheese	1 oz.	4g
Flounder, baked	3.5 oz.	30g
Frankfurter	2 oz.	7g
Hummus	1 Cup	12g
Kidney Beans	1/2 Cup	8g
Milk, 1% fat	1 Cup	8g
Milk, 2% fat	1 Cup	8g
Milk, skim	1 Cup	8g
Milk, whole	1 Cup	8g
Mozzarella cheese	1 oz.	6g
Mutton, (lamb)	100g	17g
Pasta, cooked	1 Cup	5g
Peanut Butter	1 Tbsp	4g
Pork ribs, lean broiled	3.5 oz.	29g
Pork Roast	3 oz.	21g

Rice, brown, cooked	1 Cup	5g
Rice, white, cooked	1 Cup	4g
Sausage, cooked	1 Patty	5g
Shrimp, cooked	12 Large	17g
Snapper	3 oz.	21g
Soymilk	1 Cup	6g
Spanish Rice	1 Cup	4g
Tofu	100g	9g
Tortilla Corn	1	2g
Tuna in oil	3oz.	24g
Turkey, light meat	3oz.	28g
Yogurt, whole milk	8oz.	7g
Black beans, boiled	1 Cup	15g

Successful people who are leaders many times can be more of a challenge to teach. It's harder for them to listen to someone share the basics of a simple weight loss plan. They should remember that the way they became a success in business is the same way they will become a success in losing weight. Back to basics!

Maintaining Your New Weight

The frustration of the repetitive cycle of losing and gaining weight is the worst of all frustrations. This can become a memory by developing the habits set forth in this book.

You might try counting the people who lose weight and then gain the weight back after losing it and never find an end. Don't feel bad, I never met anybody who knew how to maintain their weight. I never heard a lecture on it, read a book or journal, or heard a discussion on it at medical conferences.

This cycle should stop for you when you've finished this chapter you will understand and know how to maintain where you're happy for the rest of your life with no more up and downs.

Many people think what they did was wrong and go from one doctor or clinic to another looking for the answer with frustration.

With all that said, it's time now to get to the core of the problem which can be said in one word, habits. Habits got us where we are today and habits are going to get us where we want to go. Don't worry we're going to have fun with this boring subject or at least try!

When you hear the word habit, most of us think of smoking which some people may never quit no matter what, this holds true for eating habits which some will never change or even consider that a habit can be a powerful tool if cultivated, developed and applied in many areas of your life which could have good or bad outcome.

Steve

Bare with me now because this relates to me. Steve, one of my room-mates in college was studying pre-law while I was studying pre-med did something that changed my life and my grades.

Everyday without exception, he was in our room from 3:00 to 5:00 studying, he never quit before 5:00, not even by a few minutes. During the two hours he would dedicate himself to go over the material continuously till time was up. After watching him for a few months I joined him with the two hour study time, mine being chemistry which my grades were usually a low B. After sticking with a strict study time each day my grades went up to all A's. Thanks to Steve for being my best example of a good habit to this day.

When I see a patient for the first time, I say, "You are not going to be on a diet, instead you'll learn how to eat less of the major problem foods which are in front of us just about every time we eat ... bread, potatoes and sweets. We are never going to stop eating these problem foods at anytime. If you do you will fail for sure as the feeling of being deprived will overtake you and you will gain more weight back than before you started. Every meal without exception, eat less of the bread, potatoes and when finished eat even less of the dessert.

Example:

At breakfast eat eggs, bacon and one slice of toast instead of two. At noon take the top off of your sandwich, and throw it away. If you do this for thirty days then you will have thrown away sixty pieces of bread (throwing away two a day for thirty days is sixty).

People usually fail when they don't stick to the plan. The plan is to remove one slice of bread from a sandwich before you eat it then eliminate two thirds of your potatoes, cut down on sweets. Every meal three times a day you follow the plan.

Most people should lose between eight and twelve pounds the first month following this plan. On returning most patients say they feel great and it was not hard at all to do. Then I advise them to increase their protein which stimulates the hormone (glucagon to lose weight which is from the alpha cells in the pancreas). When eating too much bread, potatoes and sweets, insulin is up which creates the fat problem.

The next visit I ask, "Do you feel like your getting in the habit of what we discussed on your last visit?" Usually the patient will say it's getting easier everyday thinking they're going to make it. I also explain what I do at every meal I eat.

My professor said to me years ago, "It will take you 60 to 90 days to develop a habit and if within 30 days you eat a sandwich with both pieces of bread your 60 days will start over from that minute. After 60 days everything should become automatic and natural with no thinking, and you will have mastered maintenance forever.

The goal is for us to get to the point that we don't think about what to eat or not eat, just do it because it has become natural to eat less of the bread, potatoes, sweets or desserts.

I tell my patients, "I want for you to know how wonderful it is to not ever think of food again and to be your ideal weight. When the habits develop it will not require any thinking just like your old habits didn't require any thought."

When you are trim and staying there,
someone will ask you,
"Please tell me what you do!"
Answer like this:
It's not what I do
It's what I did do
When I didn't have to do
Now I don't have to do
What I did do and
Don't do now!
Eating has become automatic with very
little thinking.

Have Fun

Are you serious, lose weight at fast food places? Sure can if you know how. Fast food places are in Hong Kong, Tokyo, New York, London, Paris and all over the world. People in all walks of life, executives, business men and ladies, sometimes are in a fast food place because they have to be.

Have fun by knowing how to lose weight.

Example:
1. Order a Big Mac, take the top bun off and the middle piece of bread and that takes care of a sudden rise in blood sugar-the 2 pieces of meat, cheese, lettuce and to-mato helps us lose as the protein makes the hormone to lose weight go up, and lettuce and tomato being complex carbs slow down digestion.

2. The mixed salad with chicken on top, raw salad has fiber slowing down digestion and prevents blood sugar from rising rapidly, helping weight loss and the meat makes the other hormone go up helping weigh loss.

3. Chicken Nuggets with the sauce you like, just peel a lit-tle of the breading off, it's mostly protein, which helps with weight loss.

4. Sausage, egg and cheese biscuit. Take the top piece of bread off and peel the edges of the bottom piece off.

5. When having a steak the protein stimulates the pancre-as to raise the hormone to lose weight. Ask your server to bring you a few potato skins with cheese instead of the baked potato. The skin doesn't elevate blood sugar helping weight loss and the cheese helps too.

The salad that came with your dinner also helps, because fresh vegetables are complex carbs containing fiber, slowing down digestion, and helping weight loss also. You may be the only one there knowing how to lose weight.

Years ago the football coach from Oklahoma was in Dallas and had an appointment with H.L. Hunt who was one of the richest men during his time. In his office after a nice visit, Mr. Hunt asked the coach if he would like to have lunch with him and he promptly said, "Yes, thank you." Then Mr. Hunt pulled his desk drawer open, pulled out a brown sack with a peanut butter and jelly sandwich which he cut in half and said, "You'll have to excuse this, my wife was still in bed when I left this morning and I had to make this myself."

Isn't it great when a man like that was still down to earth? I carry a brown sack to my office every day and have since grade school and when eating out, I enjoy it more than most because it's a treat for me.

Teens

Whether they want to admit it or not, anyone who is overweight wants to lose weight, but this desire is particularly heightened in teens, especially teen girls. However wrong, society and their peers tend to attach more stigma to overweight teen girls.

If you've ever reared a teenager you know how sensitive they can be, so how you approach the weight issue is important. They'll be turned off immediately with the lecturing, condemnation, or reprimanding.

A statement such as, "My jeans are too tight" may be the only opening you need. This is your opportunity to bring up a healthy life style. You might want to say to them, "If I knew a doctor who helped teens get to their healthiest weight without depriving themselves of the foods they love, would you be interested in talking with him? He teaches you how you can lose weight by modifying how you eat the foods you love like hamburgers, fries or pizza. Things as simple as removing the top part of the bun on the burger, eating more meat and cheese on thin crust pizza, half of the fries and sweets, cutting soft drinks in half and drinking more water with these new eating habits which will cause dramatic weight loss."

We all know sometimes when something is said to a teen about anything they tune us out, look down or the other way. It's done to parents and me when they are brought in for help. There is help. The answer is simple which I discovered coincidentally observing a patient in their home. Teens themselves are the answer as they will listen and do what another teen says if they respect and admire that teen.

Example:
A young man, about fifteen years of age, having trouble with his swing while attempting to hit that baseball will listen

to pointers from a fellow team mate because he wants to be like the older teen that he respects. Usually there are no questions asked, they just tell them what to do and it is done. So if a teenage friend or older sibling says, "Start throwing some of that bread away on the sandwich or hamburger, eat a few of your fries, switch to diet drinks and get off the candy kick." With this simple plan the teens from twelve to sixteen will trim up and have healthier habits for the rest of their life.

The obesity epidemic our country is having has become a national concern and recently prompted republicans and democrats to have a forum to see if anything could be done to remedy this situation. Many things were discussed about prevention, cost, utilization, research, education, treatment, taxation and discrimination. Although everyone attending was concerned, very few thought there would be a medical cure for obesity anytime in the near future and did not have any current solutions.

I know the answer is all around us everywhere we look. Today's teens could be the first generation NOT to have the obesity problem. If today's teens were taught and learned the basics, a new healthy trim America is in the future. All we need is one teen in every home who knows what to do and all the food companies would join in providing the healthy food and snacks. Prove this to yourself or several friends who have teens with weight problems and you will be just amazed as I have been.

Your Stimulus Package

We all know about the Economic Stimulus package. Now learn about the health and weight loss stimulus package that is in place and being given now to everybody in America young, old, rich or poor.

The obesity epidemic is not only here, but has become global and other countries are experiencing it also. It is not only in the process of being stopped, but reversed and some will be under their ideal weight instead of way above.

This stimulus is not from the government, doctors, clinics or medical institutions, but from my new unknown, unrecognized heroes of the major and minor food distributing and manufacturing companies.

These people have studied hard with long hours of reading medical books, journals, reprints and everything they can get their hands on concerning food ingredients, what they do in our body for weight management and better health. Do you know how I know their studying? Because their reading the same things I'm reading.

Learn what these companies have done as well as myself and when shopping apply it by looking at protein, carbs, sugar and fiber content and follow their lead.

They are increasing protein, vitamins and fiber in their foods and decreasing carbs and sugars. This is perfect for better health and weight loss, my work is actually becoming easier. Patients are daily telling me about a new food, just last week a lady said, "I've found the cure for these chocolate cravings which is the Jell-O no sugar chocolate pudding."

My nurse was going shopping that day and I asked her to pick up some. Another patient told me, " I look at protein on the label and fiber first and if up, it goes in the basket."

Now while helping people lose weight patients are constantly telling family and friends which also spread the word. Recently a patient called me from California and said her mother, sister and a couple others were doing it. In time this will cover the country.

Now you know about one of the greatest things in our country happening before any news commentator or stations knows.

SEE IT

LEARN IT

TEACH IT

My Dream

An obese poor lady who is raising 4 or 5 children that were dumped on her to raise is going through a super center buying food and starting with 6 loaves of bread which has been fixed with some protein, low carbohydrates and extra fiber. On the next aisle the cereal is also fixed as well as the cookies. Everything else in the store is fixed. Thanks to the giants in our food companies and to everyone doing their part.

This poor lady who knows nothing about what different foods do to her body, never seen a doctor or a clinic or read anything about weight loss or health will be taken care of. She will begin to lose weight each month and even though not understanding about causes of diabetes, high blood pressure or heart conditions, she will have less chance of suffering from any of these health problems. Instead she'll be healthier with more energy and it didn't matter that she didn't have any money.

With all that's on this lady in taking care of others problems, it doesn't leave any time for herself and impossible to go to a clinic or weight loss doctor which she could not afford if she had the time. Nobody knows it, but I bet she dreams of having the weight off with a trim look. Food companies with their new methods of preparing foods are making her dreams become real and mine also with many others being trim.

Final Thoughts

If you are not satisfied with past experiences or your present situation then consider doing what I have done for many years and it works under stress, traveling, at work or while eating on the run.

When you take control of this part of your life you will become the person you've always wanted to be with not only your new look, but believing in yourself and enjoying your new life and looking forward to the future.

You can be one of the few who have mastered weight control.

VITAMIN RESOURCES

Vitamins Now May Prevent Chemo Later

The information here is for those who would like to know more about vitamins, supplements and minerals. This should not take the place of advice or treatment you are presently receiving. Before doing anything you read here, consult with your present physician or a qualified health professional.

Vitamins and minerals make our immune system stronger and in that fashion helps prevent cancer and many other diseases so we need it working at peak performance.

It's good to know about each vitamin as they all work together in harmony to keep us healthier and living a longer, fuller life with more energy.

Everyone wants to stay young as they can for as long as possible, have more energy, less sickness, less doctor visits and hospital stays. Years ago there was not much in the medical literature about vitamins, but now it's in most literature including the newspapers.

For example, countries that have low selenium levels in the soil have more cancer. Lycopene found in tomatoes is low in the blood of patients with cancer of the pancreas and prostate. Vitamin C blood levels are low in patients with cancer of the stomach and we could go on and on.

The foods we eat many times don't have what we need as farm soil has been used over and over for many years and many times over fertilized. We need to look at vitamins and minerals in food we didn't get at the table.

Someday, I hope our medical schools will have a course on disease prevention as well as how to treat a particular one, this will happen it's just a matter of time.

Vitamin A

Vitamin A is a naturally occurring molecule called retinoid which helps build and maintain a strong and effective immune system.

It is found in carrots, spinach, carrot juice, sweet potatoes, pumpkin, mangos, beat greens, turnip greens, tuna and buttermilk squash to name a few.

A deficiency could manifest itself with night blindness and hard to recover vision after facing headlights of an oncoming car. Also difficulty in maintaining your balance, poor appetite, abnormal color vision, dry eyes, taste and smell difficulties.

Vitamin A is fat soluble and taking it with a food that has some fat in it is necessary for absorption. Some diseases may increase the need for more which are cancer, pneumonia, TB, nephritis, prostate disease and urinary infections.

This vitamin can be toxic in high doses of 10,000 international units or above and women in the childbearing age should consult with their doctor before taking. The daily value is 5,000 international units. I do not recommend the supplement but adequate amount of Vitamin A can be obtained from eating fruits and vegetables loaded with beta-carotene which our body will turn into Vitamin A to supply our needs.

Vitamin B - Complex

Did you know you can buy a pill over the counter that is a tranquilizer, mood elevator, stress reducer, increases learning ability and sleeping pill all in one? If someday you are stressed out, irritable or down right disgusted about something, try taking a B - Complex (all the different B's in it). One before going to bed after a late party and again in the AM helps tremendously.

I have personally seen many patients through the years get good results in bringing down cholesterol with one B - Complex daily and two odor free garlic tablets. The garlic tablets should be taken with food or after eating, which will effect the liver functions better. I personally do this daily and have for years.

You might want to try this, at that time of the month or PMS, take 200mg of vitamin B-6 each day for a week before menses and during menses. At a banquet, a lady across the table we were at said, "Thanks doc for suggestions of B-6" and her husband spoke up and said, "Yea doc, thanks a lot!"

B6 also helps in the making of T- Cells and white blood cells that battle infection. In this fashion our immune system is better prepared.

If over 40 you might want to get a B - 12 injection monthly for more energy (I do).

Dosage - One B - Complex daily.

Vitamin C

If I could only take one vitamin a day, it would be Vitamin C because it protects us in not one but many diversified ways.

Years ago, sailors in the English Navy were coming down with an unknown disease with loss of appetite, fatigue, extreme weakness, bleeding under the skin, in joints and gums around the teeth. They found that by putting bushels of limes on the ship for the men to eat daily stopped the disease. You might have heard that the sailors in the British Navy are some times called limeys. The extreme Vitamin C deficiency was the culprit and it was called scurvy.

You wouldn't think scurvy would even occur here and especially in a millionaires home with a maid and all the luxuries.

A friend asked me to examine his 12 year old son who was pale, listless, weak, no energy and no interest in anything. The problem was the maid was trying to be extra clean and was boiling his orange juice, which completely destroyed the Vitamin C. He had scurvy and had dramatic and quick results by taking Vitamin C and proper juices. It's amazing how sometimes simple can handle a serious problem.

Our main priority is doing all we can to prevent cancer, infections and other diseases by keeping our immune system strong and at it's best to do what it is made to do as our defense. All the vitamins have a part here with the main one being Vitamin C which is an antioxidant.

Remember about the free radicals from the oxidation process and the damage done to our cells?

Vitamin C leads here to prevent this as much as possible while slowing the activity of viruses and bacteria and lessens the symptoms of allergies and asthma.

The National Cancer Institute thinks the evidence is strong enough to warrant a high Vitamin C diet.

Dosage 1,000 to 2,000 mg a day (taken with food or after meals).

If history of stomach ulcers or problems check with your physician before taking.

Vitamin D

In the April of 2005 Journal of Renal and Urology News which is a world review, the headline was, "Vitamin D may cut prostate cancer risk and be another potential strategy." When sunlight hits the skin Vitamin D is formed and may possibly help prevent other tumors.

It also aids in the treatment of osteoporosis making bones stronger and added as a supplement in Crohn's disease.

I think this is just the beginning and further research with sunlight may be very rewarding.

Vitamin E

Do you have to prop your feet up at the end of the day because of leg cramps? I had that problem for several years over thirty to be exact. I took 400-800 units of Vitamin E and after 4-6 months the cramps went away and I have not had any leg cramps for thirty years now. Don't give up, it took a few months to have its effect! I know of others who have also done this.

Did you know more doctors take Vitamin E than any other vitamin? I think it helps by making our blood vessels cleaner and allows more oxygen to different areas with better blood flow.

A Harvard study of 87,000 nurses on Vitamin E for eight years had a 36% lower risk of major coronary disease.

Another thing that it does is boost the immune system, slows aging, anti-cancer, fibrocystic disease of the breast, PMS, would heal with less scarring and help in the treatment of Lupus.

Dosage 400-800 units daily.

Calcium

If we fall or have an accident we want our bones as strong as possible. Calcium working with Vitamin D helps absorb better and the result is we have less osteoporosis which is brittle bones.

Some studies have shown there is a higher incidence of hypertension associated with low calcium and high sodium. Improvement was seen with calcium supplements.

There have been some studies showing where calcium helps prevent colon cancer. Dairy products also help and here we go again, sunlight does too. Remember the Vitamin D helping prevent cancer as we discussed which is formed when the sun hits the skin.

Calcium also gives us more energy, helps in muscle contractions and relaxation (heart also).

Here is a secret. Sometimes I take a B - Complex and a Calcium pill for a better night sleep.

Magnesium

Did you know the test to measure the blood level of magnesium is one of the first test heart doctors order if they think angina of coronary blockage is present?

Since magnesium aids with muscle spasm by relaxation and affects blood vessel tone this is the reason the test is ordered. Every time your heart beats, it contracts then relaxes, contracts then relaxes. Cal - Mag which is a combination of the two together and comes in a pill form.

Magnesium is also low in Autism and they need B - 6 too.

Dosage 500 - 750 mg daily.

RECIPES

Barbecued Ginger Chicken

Ingredients

2 tablespoons brown sugar, packed

1/4 cup ketchup

1 tablespoon Worcestershire sauce

1 tablespoon vinegar

1 teaspoon grated gingerroot

1/4 teaspoon dried red pepper flakes (optional)

4 skinless chicken breasts, rinsed, and patted dry

Directions

Preheat broiler or grill.

In a small mixing bowl, combine all ingredients except chicken and mix well.

Reserve 1/4 cup sauce in a separate dish.

Coat a broiler rack and pan with cooking spray and add chicken.

Broil 12-15 minutes or until no longer pink in center, turning and basting occasionally with sauce.

Remove from broiler and spoon reserved 1/4 cup sauce evenly over all.

Nutrition Facts

Recipe makes 4 servings.

Serving size 1 (162g)

Calories 207

Calories from Fat 38 (18%)

Amount per serving %DV

Total Fat 4.3g 6%

Saturated Fat 1.1g 5%

Trans Fat 0.1g

Cholesterol 95mg 31%

Dietary Fiber 0.1g

Sugars 13.9g

Protein 26.3g 52%

Herbed Beef Tenderloin

Ingredients

3 - 4 lbs. beef tenderloin

3 garlic cloves, minced

2 teaspoons fresh rosemary, finely minced

2 teaspoons fresh thyme, finely minced

Directions

Rub garlic cloves onto tenderloin and season with minced herbs.

Let it sit for 20 minutes.

Preheat oven to 475 degrees F. with the broiler pan in the oven.

Place tenderloin on pan, put into oven and reduce heat to 375 degrees F for 20 minutes.

Reduce heat again to 325 degrees F for 20 minutes.

Remove from oven and tent with foil. Let meat "rest" for 20 minutes, slice for serving.

Nutrition Facts

Recipe makes 6 servings.

Serving size 1 (228g)

Calories 662

Calories from Fat 413 (62%)

Amount per serving %DV

Total Fat 45.9g 70%

Saturated Fat 18.0g 90%

Monounsaturated Fat 18.8g

Polyunsaturated Fat 1.8g

Trans Fat 0.0g

Cholesterol 194mg 64%

Sodium 134mg 5%

Potassium 843mg 24%

Total Carbohydrate 0.6g 0%

Dietary Fiber 0.1g

Sugars 0.0g

Protein 57.4g 114%

Citrus Chili Shrimp

Ingredients

1/3 cup olive oil

1/3 cup orange juice, divided

2 tablespoons fresh lime juice (one half of a lime)

1/2 teaspoon salt

1/4 teaspoon red pepper flakes

1/4 teaspoon chili powder

1/4 teaspoon ground cumin

1-1/2 lbs medium shrimp, peeled and deveined

1 tablespoon olive oil

1 tablespoon butter

Directions

In a medium bowl, mix 1/3 cup olive oil, 3 TB orange juice, half of the lime juice, salt red pepper, chili powder and cumin. Add shrimp and marinade for 10 minutes.

In a large skillet over medium high heat, melt butter with tablespoon of olive oil. With a slotted spoon remove shrimp from marinade; reserve marinade for later use. Add shrimp to skillet. Cook for about 4 minutes, until no longer pink and just cooked through. Transfer shrimp to a plate.

Add reserved marinade to skillet. Add remaining orange and lime juices. Bring to a full boil, boil one minute, pour over remaining shrimp on plate.

Serve immediately.

Nutrition Facts
Recipe makes 4 servings.

Serving size 1 (224g)

Calories 407

Calories from Fat 245 (60%)

Garlic and Maple Salmon

Ingredients

1/4 cup maple syrup

2 tablespoon soy sauce

1 garlic clove, minced

1/4 teaspoon garlic salt

1/8 teaspoon ground black pepper

4 skinless chicken breasts, rinsed, and patted dry

Directions

In a small mixing bowl, combine all ingredients except salmon, mix well.

Place salmon in a shallow glass baking dish, and coat with the maple syrup mixture. Cover the dish and marinate salmon in the refrigerator for 30 minutes, turning once.

Preheat oven to 400 degrees F.

Place the baking dish in the preheated oven, and bake salmon uncovered 20 minutes, or until easily flaked with a fork.

Nutrition Facts

Recipe makes 4 servings.

Serving size 1 (149g)

Calories 190

Calories from Fat 35 (18%)

Amount per serving %DV

Total Fat 4.0g 6%

Monounsaturated Fat 1.1g

Polyunsaturated Fat 1.6g

Trans Fat 0.10

Cholesterol 58mg 19%

Dietary Fiber 0.1g

Protein 23.6g 47%

Stuffed Ricotta Chicken

Ingredients

6 chicken legs with thighs attached

1/2 ounce butter, melted

2 slices bacon, finely chopped

1 tablespoon olive oil

1 small onion, diced

1 clove garlic, crushed

8 ounces ricotta cheese

1 egg, beaten

2 tablespoons freshly grated parmesan cheese

1 cup breadcrumbs

1/4 cup fresh parsley, chopped

2 tablespoons fresh chives, chopped

Directions

Finely chop bacon and fry until crisp, remove when cooked and set aside.

In the same pan, heat the oil and cook the garlic and onion until soft.

Put ricotta cheese, egg, parmesan, breadcrumbs, parsley, chives, tarragon, bacon, onion, garlic and nutmeg in a large bowl. Mix together.

Preheat oven to 350 degrees F.

Using your fingers, ease the skin away from the thigh and leg of the chicken, being careful not to pierce the skin.

Gently push stuffing mixture evenly under the skin. Draw skin back over the stuffing. Place the chicken in a lightly oiled, shallow roasting pan.

Brush chicken with melted butter.

Roast for 45 min., until chicken is cooked through.

Remove from oven and allow to sit for 5 minutes before serving.

Nutrition Facts

Recipe makes 6 servings.

Serving size 1 (263g)

Calories 554

Calories from Fat 318 (57%)

Amount per serving %DV

Total Fat 35.4g 54%

Saturated Fat 12.4g 62%

Monounsaturated Fat 12.9g

Polyunsaturated Fat 6.8g

Trans Fat 0.2g

Cholesterol 205mg 68%

Sodium 413mg 17%

Sweet Paprika Salmon

Ingredients

2 red peppers

2 tablespoons extra virgin olive oil, plus extra for grilling and greasing

1 teaspoon paprika

Salt & Pepper to taste

6 salmon fillets, skin on, about 7oz each

Dressing

2 tablespoons olive oil

1 tablespoon lemon juice or red wine vinegar

1 tablespoon honey

To serve

9 ounces salad greens

1 tablespoon capers, rinsed and drained

Directions

Preheat oven to 425 degrees F.

Place the peppers onto a baking sheet and drizzle with olive oil. Transfer to the oven and roast for 20 minutes, or until scorched in places. Place the peppers into a bowl, cover with plastic wrap and set aside.

Place a good solid baking sheet into the oven to heat up for about three minutes.

In a bowl, mix together the olive oil, paprika, salt and pepper. Brush this spiced oil all over the salmon.

Lightly oil the hot baking sheet and place salmon onto it, skin side down. Bake for 10-12 minutes, or until the salmon is cooked but still pink inside.

When the peppers are cool enough to handle, peel skin off and cut the flesh into strips, discarding the core and seeds.

For the dressing, whisk all the dressing ingredients together in a bowl until slightly thickened. Place the salad leaves into a bowl, drizzle over the dressing and stir to coat the leaves.

To serve, place the salad onto serving plates and top with the salmon, skin side up.

Arrange the pepper strips and capers on top of salmon.

Nutrition Facts

Recipe makes 4 servings.

Serving size 1 (621g)

Calories 704

Calories from Fat 272 (38%)

Amount per serving %DV

Total Fat 30.3g 46%

Saturated Fat 4.6g 22%

Monounsaturated Fat 14.3g

Spicy Rib Eye

Ingredients

1/2 cup butter, melted

1/4 cup lemon juice

1/4 cup ketchup

2 tablespoons Worcestershire sauce

2 tablespoons olive oil

2 tablespoons cider vinegar

4 garlic cloves, minced

1 teaspoon salt

1 teaspoon sugar

1/2 teaspoon hot pepper sauce

1 dash cayenne pepper

6 (12 ounce) rib eye steaks (about 1 inch thick and 12 oz. each

Directions

In a large re-sealable bag, combine the first 11 ingredients. Add the steaks. Seal bag and turn to coat; refrigerate for 6 hours or over night.

Drain and discard marinade. Grill steaks uncovered over medium heat for 4-5 minutes on each side or until the meat reaches desired doneness. (for medium rare meat thermometer should read 145, medium 160, well done 170.

Nutrition Facts

Recipe makes 6 servings.

Serving size 1 (398g)

Calories 1130

Calories from Fat 854 (75%)

Amount per serving %DV

Total Fat 95.0g 146%

Saturated Fat 41g 204%

Monounsaturated Fat 39.93g

Polyunsaturated Fat 3.7g

Trans Fat 0.0g

Cholesterol 272mg 90%

Tangy Garlic Steak

Ingredients

4 pounds beef sirloin steaks, at least 3/4 inch thick

1 (16 ounce) bottle Italian salad dressing

2 tablespoons Worcestershire sauce

2 tablespoons minced garlic

1 teaspoon olive oil

Salt and pepper to taste

Directions

Score the steaks lightly on both sides using a sharp knife. Place in a shallow baking dish. Pour the Italian dressing and Worcestershire sauce over them, and sprinkle with garlic. Rub the marinade into the steaks using the back of a spoon or fork. Turn steaks over, and repeat on the other side. Marinate in the refrigerator for 2 to 24 hours.

Preheat a grill to medium - high heat. Oil the grate lightly with a paper towel dipped in olive oil.

Grill steaks for about 6 minutes per side, or to desired doneness. Season with salt and pepper to taste before serving.

Ginger Steak

Ingredients

  4 (8 ounce) beef sirloin steaks, at least 3/4 inch thick

  2 tablespoons soy sauce

  1 tablespoons ground ginger

  1 teaspoon lemon juice

  1/2 teaspoon salt

  1 teaspoon pepper

  1 teaspoon dried basil

  1 tablespoon prepared yellow mustard

Directions

  Preheat the oven broiler.

  In a small bowl, mix together the soy sauce, ginger, salt, pepper, basil, mustard and lemon juice until smooth. Place the steaks on a broiling pan, and pour 1/4 of the mixture over each steak. Massage into the meat.

  Broil steaks for 5 minutes, then turn over and cook to your desired degree of doneness.

Ginger Salmon

Ingredients

    2 teaspoons olive oil

    1 tablespoon honey

    1 tablespoon Dijon mustard

    2 teaspoons grated fresh ginger

    1 pound salmon fillets

Directions

Preheat oven to 350 degrees F (175 degrees C).

In a small bowl, blend olive oil, honey, Dijon mustard and ginger.

Brush salmon fillets evenly with the olive oil mixture. Place in a medium baking dish. Bake 15 to 20 minutes in the preheated oven, until fish flakes easily with a fork.

Goat Cheese Salmon

Ingredients

4 salmon fillets

1/2 cup herbed goat cheese

1/4 cup prepared Dijon mustard mayonnaise

Salt and pepper to taste

Directions

Preheat oven to 350 degrees F (175 degrees C). Lightly grease a large baking dish.

Arrange the salmon fillets in the baking dish.

Make small incisions in each fillet, and stuff with equal amounts of the herbed goat cheese.

Spread equal amounts prepared Dijon mustard mayonnaise, blend over each fillet. Season with salt and pepper to taste.

Bake salmon for 15 minutes in preheated oven, or until easily flaked with a fork.

Lemon Rosemary Salmon

Ingredients

2 salmon fillets, bones and skin removed

1 lemon, thinly sliced

Coarse salt to taste

4 sprigs, fresh rosemary

1 teaspoon olive oil

Salt and pepper to taste

Directions

Preheat oven to 400 degrees F (200 degrees C)

Arrange half the lemon slices in a single layer in a baking dish. Layer with 2 sprigs rosemary, top with salmon fillets. Sprinkle salmon with salt, layer with remaining rosemary sprigs, and top with remaining lemon slices. Drizzle with olive oil.

Bake for 20 minutes in the preheated oven, or until fish is easily flaked with a fork.

Creole Pan-Fried Flat Iron Steak

Ingredients

2 pounds flat iron steak

1 tablespoon hot pepper sauce

2 tablespoons lime juice

2 teaspoons garlic salt

1/8 teaspoon salt

1/8 teaspoon ground black pepper

2 - 1/4 teaspoons blackened seasoning

1/2 cup butter

1/2 cup water

Directions

Heat a skillet over medium heat. Season the steak with hot pepper sauce. Sprinkle or mist with a little lime juice and season lightly with just a portion of the garlic salt, salt, black pepper and blackened seasoning.

Place the steak in the pan and cover with lid. Cook for about 20 minutes, or to your desired degree of doneness, turning and adding more seasoning every 5 minutes.

Remove steaks to a serving platter and keep warm. Stir butter and water into pan, removing any browned bits from the bottom to make a gravy. Season with additional garlic salt, salt and pepper to taste. Serve steaks with gravy drizzled over them.

Jalapeno Steak

Ingredients

4 jalapeno peppers, stemmed

4 garlic cloves, peeled

2 tablespoons Worcestershire sauce

1-1/2 teaspoons cracked black pepper

1 tablespoon coarse salt

1/4 cup lime juice

1 tablespoon dried oregano

1-1/2 pounds top sirloin steak

Directions

Combine jalapenos, garlic, pepper, salt, lime juice and oregano in a blender. Blend until smooth.

Place steak in a shallow pan or large re-sealable plastic bag. Pour jalapeno marinade over steak, turn to coat. Cover pan or seal bag.

Marinate in the refrigerator 8 hours or overnight.

Preheat an outdoor grill for high heat, and lightly oil the grill grate.

Drain and discard marinade. Grill steak 5 minutes per side, or to desired doneness.

Citrus Orange Roughy

Ingredients

1/2 cup dry bread crumbs

3/4 teaspoon salt

1/2 cup orange juice

2 tablespoons reduced - sodium soy sauce

1 tablespoon butter or stick margarine, melted

1/2 teaspoon lemon juice

4 (6 ounce) fillets Orange Roughy

Directions

In a shallow bowl, combine bread crumbs and salt.

In another shallow bowl, combine the orange juice, soy sauce, butter, oil and lemon juice.

Dip the fillets into orange juice mixture, then coat with crumb mixture.

Place in a 13 inch x 9 inch x 2 inch baking dish coated with nonstick cooking spray.

Bake, uncovered at 450 degrees F for 15 to 18 minutes or until fish flakes easily with a fork.

Zesty Tilapia with Mushrooms

Ingredients

1 ounce dried porcini mushrooms

2 tablespoons butter

2 (4 ounce) fillets tilapia, halved

kosher salt to taste

ground black pepper to taste

1 tablespoon lemon zest

2 limes, juiced

2 green onions, chopped

Directions

Place dried porcini mushrooms in a small bowl with enough warm water to cover. Soak 20 minutes, or until rehydrated, and chop.

Melt 1 tablespoon butter in a medium skillet over medium heat. Place tilapia in the skillet, and season with kosher salt and pepper. Sprinkle with 1/2 the lemon zest. Pour half the lime juice over the tilapia, and continue cooking for 5 minutes.

Flip the tilapia, and season with kosher salt and pepper. Sprinkle with remaining lemon zest, and cover with remaining lime juice. Stir remaining butter, green onions, and porcini mushrooms into the skillet. Continue cooking 5 minutes, or until fish is easily flaked with a fork.

Easy Baked Chicken Cordon Bleu

Ingredients

6 skinless, boneless chicken breast halves - pounded to 1/2 inch thickness

6 string cheese sticks

6 slices ham

1/2 cup butter, melted

1 cup seasoned dry bread crumbs

toothpicks

Directions

Preheat oven to 350 degrees F.

Lay out pounded chicken breasts on a clean surface. Place a slice of ham on each piece, then one stick of cheese. Roll the chicken up around the cheese and ham, and secure with toothpicks. Dip each roll in melted butter then roll in bread crumbs. Place in a shallow baking dish.

Bake for 40 minutes in the preheated oven, or until chicken is browned and juices run clear.

Easy Italian Chicken

Ingredients

4 (8 ounce) beef sirloin steaks, at least 3/4 inch thick

2 tablespoons soy sauce

1 tablespoons ground ginger

1 teaspoon lemon juice

1/2 teaspoon salt

1 teaspoon pepper

1 teaspoon dried basil

1 tablespoon prepared yellow mustard

Directions

Preheat the oven broiler.

In a small bowl, mix together the soy sauce, ginger, salt, pepper, basil, mustard and lemon juice until smooth. Place the steaks on a broiling pan, and pour 1/4 of the mixture over each steak. Massage into the meat.

Broil steaks for 5 minutes, then turn over and cook to your desired degree of doneness.

Easy Baked Chicken Cordon Bleu

Ingredients

6 skinless, boneless chicken breast halves - pounded to 1/2 inch thickness

6 string cheese sticks

6 slices ham

1/2 cup butter, melted

1 cup seasoned dry bread crumbs

toothpicks

Directions

Preheat oven to 350 degrees F.

Lay out pounded chicken breasts on a clean surface. Place a slice of ham on each piece, then one stick of cheese. Roll the chicken up around the cheese and ham, and secure with toothpicks. Dip each roll in melted butter, then roll in bread crumbs. Place in a shallow baking dish.

Bake for 40 minutes in the preheated oven, or until chicken is browned and juices run clear.

Chicken Julienne

Ingredients

1 pound skinless, boneless chicken breast, cut into strips

1/2 cup butter, melted

1/2 cup all-purpose flour

2 tablespoons fresh lemon juice

Salt and pepper to taste

1 cup heavy cream

1/2 cup grated parmesan cheese

1 dash paprika, for garnish

Directions

Preheat oven to 400 degrees F (200 degrees C). Lightly grease a baking dish.

Place the butter and flour in separate shallow dishes. Dredge the chicken strips first in the flour, coating evenly, then in the butter. Place chicken in prepared baking dish.

Sprinkle with lemon juice. Add salt and pepper to taste.

Pour the heavy cream over the chicken. Sprinkle evenly with parmesan cheese, and paprika.

Bake in preheated oven until cheese melts and cream bubbles, about 20 minutes.

Seared Ahi Tuna Steaks

Ingredients

2 (5 ounce) Ahi tuna steaks

1 teaspoon kosher salt

1/4 teaspoon cayenne pepper

1/2 tablespoon butter

2 tablespoons olive oil

1 teaspoon whole peppercorns

Directions

Season the tuna steaks with salt and cayenne pepper.

Melt butter with the olive oil in a skillet over medium-high heat. Cook the peppercorns in the mixture until they soften and pop, about 5 minutes. Gently place the seasoned tuna in the skillet and cook to desired doneness. 1 - 1/2 minutes per side for rare.

Sweet Bacon Wrapped Pork Loin

Ingredients

1 (3 pound) boneless pork loin

8 slices bacon

2 tablespoons honey

2 tablespoons balsamic vinegar

2 tablespoons dry red wine

1 sweet onion, minced

1 tablespoon chopped fresh rosemary

2 tablespoons golden raisins

Salt and pepper to taste

Directions

Preheat oven to 375 degrees F (175 degrees C). Line shallow roasting pan with aluminum foil.

Season pork loin with salt and pepper. Wrap the bacon slices around the pork loin and secure with toothpicks. Preheat a large skillet over medium-high heat, then add the pork loin. Cook until golden brown on all sides, about 10 minutes, then place onto roasting pan. Stir together honey, balsamic vinegar, red wine, onion and rosemary in a small bowl, spread over pork loin.

Roast the pork loin in preheated oven for 15 minutes, then sprinkle with raisins. Continue cooking until the internal temperature of the pork loin reaches 160 degrees F (70 degrees C), about 15 minutes more. Removing from the oven, and allow to rest for 5 minutes before removing toothpicks and slicing.

Orange Soy Pork Loin

Ingredients

1 (5 pound) boneless pork loin roast

1/2 cup orange juice

1/3 cup soy sauce

1/4 tablespoons olive oil

1 tablespoon dried rosemary

1- 1/2 teaspoons chopped garlic

1 red onion, sliced

Directions

Preheat oven to 350 degrees F (175 degrees C).

In a medium bowl, stir together the orange juice, soy sauce, olive oil, red onion slices, rosemary and garlic. Place the pork roast in a baking bag, and set in a roasting pan or baking dish. Pour the orange juice mixture over the roast, making sure to coat entirely. Close the bag according to package instructions.

Bake for 2 to 2 1/2 hours in the preheated oven, until the internal temperature of the pork loin is at least 160 degrees F (70 degrees C). Remove from the oven, let stand for about 10 minutes to settle the juices. Carefully open the bag and remove the roast. Slice and serve with a little of the drippings drizzled over.

Roasted Pork Loin

Ingredients

2 pounds boneless pork loin roast

3 cloves garlic, minced

1/4 cup olive oil

1/2 cup white wine

1 sweet onion, minced

1 tablespoon chopped dried rosemary

Salt and pepper to taste

Directions

Preheat oven to 350 degrees F (175 degrees C).

Crush garlic with rosemary, salt and pepper, making a paste. Pierce meat with a sharp knife in several places and press the garlic paste into the openings. Rub the meat with the remaining garlic mixture and olive oil.

Place pork loin into oven for 2 hours, turning and basting with pan liquids. After 2 hours remove roast to platter. Heat the wine in the pan and stir to loosen browned bits of food on the bottom. Serve with pan juices.

Asian Spicy Tuna Salad

Ingredients

1 (6 ounce) can solid white tuna packed in water, drained

1 teaspoon grated fresh ginger root

1/2 teaspoon diced green chile pepper

3 tablespoons finely chopped onion

1/4 cup mayonnaise

1/4 teaspoon curry powder (optional)

1/2 teaspoon fresh lemon juice

Directions

With a fork, flake tuna into a small bowl.

Mix in ginger, pepper, chopped onion, curry powder, mayonnaise, and lemon juice.

BIBLIOGRAPHY

MILLER'S DIET TIME IS HERE FOR WEIGHT LOSS & HEALTH

Handy, RC, Chesnut CH 3rd, Gass ML, Holick MF, Leib ES, Maricic M, Watts NB.

Review of treatment modalities for postmenopausal osteoporosis.

South Med J. 2005 Oct;98(10):1000-14; quiz 1015-7,1048

Review. PMID: 16295815 (PubhMed—indexed for MEDLINE)

Wilkins CH, Birge SJ.

Prevention or osteoporotic fractures in the elderly.

AM J Med. 2005 Nov; 118(11): 1190-5. Review.

PMID:16271899 (PubMed—indexed for MEDLINE)

Ries NL, Dart RC.

New developments in antidotes.

MedClin North Am. 2005 Nov 89 (6): 1379-97. Review.

PMID: 16227068 (PubMed—indexed for MEDLINE)

Smellie WS, Wilson D, Mcnulty CA, Galloway MJ, Spikett GA, Finnigan DI, Barefoot DA, Greig MA,

RichardsJ.

Best practice in primary care pathology: Review 1.

J Clin Pathol. 2005 Oct;58 (10): 1016-24. Review.

PMID: 16093468 (PubMed-indexed for MEDLINE)

Jacobs TP, Bilezikian JP.

Clinical review: Rare cause of hypercalcemia

J Clin Ednocinal Metab. 2005 Nov; 90 (11): 6316-22

Epub 2005 Aug 30. Review

PMID: 16131579 (PubMed—indexed for MEDLINE)

Rosen CJ.

Clinical practice. Postmenopausal osteoporosis.

N Engl J Med. 2005 Aug 11; 353 (6): 595-603

Review. No abstract available.

PMID: 16093468 (PubMed - indexed for MEDLINE)

Dirge CJ.

Is vitamin A implicated in the pathophysiology of increased intracranial pressure.

Neurology. 2005 Jun 14; 64 (11)

Review. No abstract available.

PMID: 15962400 (PubMed - MEDLINE)

Austin, M.A., "Plasma Triglyceride and Coronary Heart Disease." Ateriosclerosis and Thrombosis 11 (1991): 2-14

Bjorntorp, P., et al. "The Effect of Physical Training on Insulin Production in Obesity." Metabolism 19. (1970); 631-638

Black, H.R., "High Glycemic Index Foods, Over-Eating and Obesity." Pediatrics 103. (1999): E261-E266

Chew, I., et al. "Application of Glycemic Index to Mixed Meals." American Journal of Clinical Nutrition 47. (1988): 53-56.

Bornet, F., et al. "Insulinemic and Glycemic Indexes of Six Starch-Rich Foods Taken Alone and in a Mixed Meal by Type 2 Diabetics." American Journal of Clinical Nutrition 45. (1987):588-595.

Castelli, W.P., "The Triglyceride Issue: A View From Framingham." American Heart Journal 112. (1986): 432-437

Fabry. P., and J. Tepperman. "Meal Frequency-A Possible Factor in Human Pathology." American Journal of Clinical Nutrition 23. (1970): 1059-1068.

Duimetiere, P., et al. "Relationship of Plasma Insulin to the Incidence of Myocardial Infraction and Coronary Heart Disease Mortality in a Middle Aged Population." Diabetologia 19. (1980): 205-21.

Cerami, A., "Hypothesis: Glucose as Mediator of Aging." Journal of American Geriatrics Society 33. (1985): 626-634.

Depres, J.P., et al "Hyperinsulinemia as an Independent Risk Factor for Ischemic Heart Disease." New England Journal of Medicine 334. (1996): 952-957.

Am J Cardiol. 2004 Jun 3; 93 (11A:18C-26C. Effects of lipid-altering treatment in diabetes mellitus and the metabolic syndrome.

Deedwania PC, Hunninghaka DB, Bays H.

J Gerontol A Biol Sci Med Sci 2004 Feb; 59 (2): 139-42

J Gerontol A Biol Sci Med Sci 2003 Jan; 60 (1): 133-4

Insulin resistance, affective disorders, and Alzheimer's disease: review and hypothesis.

Rasgon N, Jarvik L.

Am J Cardiol, 2003 Apr 3; 91 (17A); 24E-28E

Management of patients with diabetic hyperlipidemia.

Knopp RH, Retzlaff B, Aikawa K, Kahn SE.

Northwest Lipid Research Clinic and Department of Medicine, University of Washington School of Medicine,

Seattle 98104, USA. rhknopp@u.washington.edu

Med Clin North AM. 2004 Jul; 88 (4): 847-63, ix-x

Oral anti-diabetic agents: 2004.

Lebovitz HE.

Department of Medicine, State University of New York Health Science Center at Brooklyn, 450 Clarkson Avenue, Brooklyn, NY 11203, USA

hlebovitz@attglobal.net

Anderson, R.A., et al. "Elevated Intakes of Supplemental Chromium Improve Glucose and Insulin Variables in Individuals with Type 2 Diabetes." Diabetes 46. (1997) 1786-1791.

Jha, P. et al. "The Antioxidant Vitamins and Cardiovascular Disease." A Critical Review of Epidemiologic and Clinical Trail Data." Annals of Internal Medicine 123, (1995): 860-872.

Dis Mon. 2005 Oct.– Nov.;51 (10-11): 548-614

Hypertension: a review and rationale of treatment.

Copley JB, Rasario r.

Department of Nephrology and Hypertension, Cleveland Clinic Florida, Weston, USA

BMC. 2006 Jan 14;332 (7533) : 73-S. Epub 2005 Dec 21.

Excess risk of fatal coronary heart disease associated with diabetes in men and women; meta-analysis of 37 prospective cohort studies.

Ann Intern Med. 2003 Feb4:138 (3) : 215-29

Comment in:

Ann Intern Med. 2003 Feb4;138 (3):I-52

Ann Intern Med. 2004 Nov 16, 141(10) : 822; author reply 822-3

Screening adults for type 2 diabetes; a review of the evidence for the U.S. Preventive Services Task Force.

Harris R, Donahue K, Rathore SS, Frame P, Woolf SH, Lohr KN.

BMJ. 2003 Jun 21;326 (7403) : 1371

Newly diagnosed type 2 diabetes mellitus.

Smith SM.

Laucet. 2002 Sep 7;360 (9335) : 783-9

Diet and risk of coronary heart disease and type 2 diabetes.

Mann J.

Department of Human Nutrition, University of Otago, P.O.Box 56, Dunedin, New Zealand.

jimmann@stonebow.otago.ac.nz

American Diabetes Association. Type 2 Diabetes in Children and Adolescents. "Diabetes care 22. (200): 381-389

Norday A and others

Individual effects of saturated fatty acids and fish oil on

plasma lipids and lipoproteins in normal men.

Am J Clin Nutr 57. 634, 1993.

Rimm EB, and others.

Vitamin E consumption and the risk of coronary disease in men.

N Eng J Med. 331:1, 1993

NIH Consensus Conference

Triglyceride, high-density lipoprotein, and coronary heart disease.

JAMA 269: 505-161

Kewick A. Pawan GLS.

Calorie intake in relation to bodyweight changes in the obese.

Lancet 1956; 2: 155-161

Kee IM, Paffenbarger.

Changes in body weight and longevity.

JAMA 1992; 268: 2045-2049.

Ferranni e, Buzzigoli G, Bonadonna R,

Giorico MA, Oleggini M, Grazideli L,

Pedrinelli R, Brand L, Beniacqua S.

Insulin resistance in essential hypertension.

N Eng j Med. 1987 317; 350-357

R.D. Miller, M.D.

Rimm EB, Stamper MJ, Ascherio A, Giovannucci E, Colditz GA, Willitt

Vitamin E consumption and risk of cornary heart disease in men.

N Eng J Med. 1993;328. 1450-1456.

Wolever TMS, Jenkins DJA, Jenkins AC, Josse RG.

The glycemic index: Methodology and clinical implication.

Am J Clin Nutr, 1991; 54. 846-854.

Helmrich, S.P., et al. "Physical Activity and Reduced Occurrence of Non-Insulin Dependent Diabetes Melitus."

New England Journal of Medicine 325. (1991): 147-152

Heshka, S., et al. "Weight Loss With Self-Help Compared with Structured

Commercial Program." JAMA 289. (1991).

Am J Cardiol. 2004 Jun 3; 93 (11A) : 27C-31C

Strategies in ongoing clinical trials to reduce cardiovascular disease in patients with diabetes mellitus and insulin resistance.

Mazzone T.

Department of Medicine, University of Illinois, Chicago, USA, tmazzone@uic.edu

Geriatrics. 2004 April; 59 (4) :18-24; quiz 25.

Diabetes in older adults. Overview of AGS guidelines for

treatment of diabetes mellitus in geriatric populations.

Olson DE, Norris SL.

Division of Endocrinology and Metabolism, Emery University School of Medicine, Atlanta, GA, USA.

Eliasson, B., and U. Smith.

"Insulin resistance is smokers and other long term users of nicotine." In Contemporary Endocrinology: Insulin Resistance, ed." G. Reaven and A. Law, pp. 121-136. Human Press 1999.

Gillman, M.W., A. Cupples, B.E. Millen, C. Ellison and P.A. Wolf.

Inverse association of dietary fat with development of ischemic stroke in men." JAMA278:2145-2150 (1997).

Hibbeln, J.R. and N. Salem.

Dietary polyunsaturated fatty acids and depression: When cholersterol does not satisfy." Am J Clin Nutr 62:1-9 (1995)

Laakso, M., et al. "Asymptomatic Atherosclerosis and Insulin Resistance. " Arterioscler Thromb 11. (1991):1068-1076

Kasin, S.E. et al. "Effects of Omega-3 Fish Oils on Lipid Metabolism, Glycemic Control and Blood Pressure in Type 2 Diabetic Patients." Journal od Clinical Endocrinology & Metabolism 67. (1988):1-5

Knapp, H.R., I.A.G. Reilly, P. Alessandrini and G,A, Fitgerald

R.D. Miller, M.D.

"In vivo indexes of plately and vascular function during fish oil administration in patients with atherosclerosis." N. Engl J Med 314 937-942 (1986).

Stevens, L.J., S.S. Zentall, J.L. Deck, M.L. Abate, B.A. Watkins, S.A. Watkins, S.A. Lipp, and J.R, Burgess. Essential fatty acid and metabolism in boys with attention-defit hyperactive disorders." Am J Clin Nutr 62: 761-768 (1995)

Lardinois, C.K., et al. "Polyunsaturated Fatty Acids Augment Insulin Secretion."

J Am Coll Nutr, 6. (1987): 507-523.

Kieren, M., et al. "Insulin Action in the Vasculature: Physiology and Pathophysiology." Journal of Vascular Research 38. (2001): 415-422

Laws, A. and G.M. Reaven. "Evidence for an Independent Relationship Between Insulin Resistance and Fasting HDL-Cholesterol, Triglyceride and Insulin Concentrations." Journal of Internal Medicine 231. (1992): 25-30.

Kohler, H-P. "Insulin Resistance Syndrome: Interaction with Coagulation and Fibronolysis." Swiss Med Weekly 132. (2002): 241-252.

Ludwig, D.S., et al. "High Glycemic Index Foods, Overeating and Obesity." Pediatrics 1-3. (1999): e26.

Muller, W.A., et al. "The Influence of Antecedent Diet Upon

Glucagons and Insulin Secretion." New England Journal of Medicine 285. (1971): 1450-1454.

Lorgeril, M., et al. "Mediterranean Dietary Pattern in a Randomized Trail: Prolong Survival and Possible Reduced Cancer Rate." Archives of Internal Medicine 158 (1998) 1181-1187.

Barrett AM

Is it Alzheimer's disease or something else? 10 disorders that may feature impaired memory and cognition. Postgrad Med. 2005 May; 117 (5): 47-53

Review. PMID: 15948369 (PubMed-indexed for MEDLINE)

Devereux F., Seaton A.

Diet as a risk factor for atopy and asthma. J Allergy Clin Immunol. 2005 Jun; 115 (6): 1109-17; quiz 118. Review. PMID: 15940119 (PubMed-indexed for MEDLINE)

Bischoff-Ferrari HA, Willett WC, Wong JB, Giovannucci E, Dietrich T, Dawson-Hughes B. Fracture prevention with vitamin D supplementation: a meta-analysis of randomized controlled trials. JAMA. 2005 may 11; 293 (18): 2257-64. Review. PMID: 1586381 (PubMed - indexed for MEDLINE)

Nieves JW.

Osteoporosis: the role of micronutrients. AM J Clin Nutr. 2005 May; 81 (5): 12328-12395. Review. PMID: 15781927 (PubMed—indexed for MEDLINE)

R.D. Miller, M.D.

Davies JH, Evans BA, Gregory JW.

Bone mass acquisition in healthy children. Arch Dis Child. 2005 Apr;90 (14); 373-8. Review. PMID: 1578192 (PubMed - indexed for MEDLINE)

Venning G.

Recent developments in vitamin D deficiency and muscle weakness among elderly people. BMJ. 2005 Mar 5;330 (7490); 524-6. Review. No abstract available. PMID: 15746134 (PubMed—indexed for MEDLIFE)

Am J Clin Nutr. 2005, 82 (1): 32-40.

Functional foods for coronary heart disease risk reduction: a meta-analysis using a multivariate approach.

Arch Inter Med. 2005 Jan 24; 165 (2): 150-6. Dietary fiber and blood pressure: a meta-analysis of randomized placebo-controlled trials.

J AM Diet Assoc. 2004 Jul; 104 (7); 1151-3. Clarifying inquiries. Does a high-fiber diet prevent colon cancer in at-risk patients?

J Fam Pract. 2003 Nov;52 (11) : 892-3.

Clinical inquiries. Does a high-fiber diet prevent colon cancer in at-risk patients?

Am J Clin Nutr. 2006 Apr;83 (4) : 760-6

Association between dietary fiber and serum C-reactive protein.

J Am Diet Assoc. 2005 Sept; 105 (9) : 1365-72

Dietary fiber and fat are associated with excess weight in young and middle-aged US adults. Howarth NC, Huang TT, Roberts SB, McCrory MA.

Am J Clin Nutr. 2004 Nov; 80 (5) : 1237-45.

Changes in whole-grain, bran, and cereal fiber consumption in relation to 8-Y weight gain in men.

Koh-Banerjee P. Franz M, Sampson L, Liu S, Jacobs DR Jr, Spiegelman D. Willett W. Rimm E.

Gut. 2004 Nov; 53 (11) : 1577-82.

Inhibitory actions of high fiber diet on intestinal gas transit in healthy volunteers.

Gonlachanvit S, Coleski R, Owyang C, Hasler W.

Parillo, M., et al. "A High Monosaturated-Fat / Low Carbohydrate Diet Improves Peripheral Insulin Sensitivity in Non-Insulin Dependent Diabetic Patients." Metabolism 41. (1992): 1373-1378.

Reaven, G.M. "Role of Insulin Resistance in Human Disease." Diabetes 37. (1988): 1495-1607.

N Engl J Med. 2002 Oct 24:347 (17) : 1342-9
Comment in:

R.D. Miller, M.D.

N Engl J Med. 2003 Feb 20; 348 (8) : 760-1; author reply 760-1.

Clinical practice. Initial management of glycemia in type 2 diabetes mellitus.

Ann Intern Med. 2002 Aug 20; 137 (4) : 263-72.

Comment in:

Ann Inter Med. 2002 Aug 20: 137 (4) : 288-9.

Ann Intern Med. 2003 Mar 18; 138 (6) : 517; author reply 517.

Test of glycemia for the diagnosis of type 2 diabetes mellitus.

Barr RG, Nathan DM, Meigs JB, Singer DE.

Massachusetts General Hospital, Harvard Medical School, Boston, Massachusetts 02114, USA rgb9@columbia.edu.

J Fam Practice, 2004 May; 53 (5) : 401-3

Clinical inquiries. Does screening for diabetes is at-risk patients improve long-term outcome?

H Langsjoen, P. Langsjoen, et al. "Usefulness of coenzyme Q 10 in clinical cardiology; A long term study, "Molecular Aspects of Medicine, 13(1994), 165-175.

P.H. Langsjoen, A.M. Langsjoen, "Overview of the use of CoQ 10 in cardiovascular disease," Biofactors, 9(1999). 273-284.

E. Baggio, R. Gamdini et al. "Italian multi-center study on the safety and efficacy of coenzyme Q10 as adjunctive therapy in heart failure, "Molecular Aspects of Medicine."

Stephen Sinatra, M.D., The Coenzyme Q10 Phenomenon

(Keats, 1998), 37

P.H. Langsjoen, K. Folkers, "A six year study of therapy of cardiomyopthy with coenzyme Q10. "International Journal of Tissue Reactions, 12 (1990) 169-171

Flokers, E. "Lovastatin decreases coenzyme Q levels in humans. "Proc National Academy Sci USA, 87 (1990), 8931-8934

Langsjoen, P.H., K. Flokers, et al. "Effective and safe therapy with coenzyme Q10 for cardiomyopthy." Klinscvhe Wochenschrift, 66 (1988), 583-590

Studies done on Coenzyme Q

Nordone DS, Westerberg D, Wolf D, Holt J.

Department of Family Medicine, Christiana Care Health System, Wilmington, DE, USA

Publication types; Review

PMID: 15125826 (PubMed - indexed for MEDLINE)

Am J Cariol. 2004 Jun3; 93 (11A) : 12C-17C

Dietary factors in the prevention of diabetes mellitus and coronary artery disease associated with the metabolic syndrome.

Maki KC.

Radient Develoment, Chicago, Illinois, USA

Kevinmaki@radientresearch.com

Anderson, T.J., et al. "The Effect of Cholesterol-Lowering and Antioxidant Therapy on Endothelial-Dependent Coronary Vasomotion." New England Journal of Medicine 332. (1995): 488-492.

R.D. Miller, M.D.

Med Clin North Am. 2004 Jul;88 (4) : 865-95,x
Insulin therapy in type 2 diabetes.

Davis T, Edelman SV

Section of Diabetes/Metabolism,

Veterans Affairs San Diego Health Care System

3350 La Jolla Village Drive 111G, San Diego, CA, USA

Am J Clin Nutr, 2004 Aug: 80 (2) : 257-63

Weight Management: Through lifestyle modification for the prevention and management of type 2 diabetes: rational and strategies. A statement of the American Diabetes Association, the North American Association for the Study of Obesity, and the American Society for Clinical Nutrition.

Klein S, Sheard NF, Pi-Sunyer X, Daly A, Wylie-Rosett J, Kulkarni K, Clark NG; American Diabetes Association; North American Association for the study of Obesity; American Society for Clinical Nutrition.

Division of Geriatrics and Nutritional Sciences and Center for Human Nutritional Sciences and Center for Human Nutrition, Washington University School of Medicine, St. Louis, MO, USA.

Ann Thorac Surg. 2004 Aug; 78 (2) : 471-3; Discussion 476
Comparison of bilateral thoracic artery grafting with percutaneous coronary interventions in diabetic patients.

Locker C, Mohr R, Lev-Ran O. Ureizky G, Frinerman A, Shaham Y. Shapira I.

Department of Cariothoracic Surgery, Tel Aviv Sourasky Medical C enter, 6 Tel Aviv 64239, Israel.

Assman, G., et al. "Olive Oil and the Mediterrnian diet: Implications for Health in Europe." British Journal of Nursing 6. (1997):675-677.

Bray, GA, "Low-Carbohydrates and Realities of Weight Loss," JAMA 289, (2003): 1853-1855.

Holick MF.

Sunlight and vitamin D for bone health and prevention of autoimmune diseases, cancers, and cardiovascular disease.

Am J Clin Nutr. 2004 Dec; 80 (6 Suppl): 1678S-88S. Review. PMID: 15585788 (PubMed - indexed for MEDLINE)

Sheth RD.

Metabolic concerns associated with antiepileptic medications. Neurology. 2004 Nov 23; 63 (10 Suppl 4): S249. Review, PMID: 15557547 (PubMed - indexed for MEDLINE)

Morgan TR, Mandyam S, Jamal MM.

Alcohol and hepatocellular carcinoma.

Gastroenterology. 2004 Nov; 127 (5 Suppl 1): S87-96. Review. PMID: 15508108 (PubMed– indexed for MEDLINE)

Garcia A, Zanibbi K.

R.D. Miller, M.D.

Homocysteine and cognitive function in elderly people. CMAJ 2004 Oct 12; 171 (8): 897-804. Review. PMID: 1547763 (PubMed—indexed for MEDLINE)

Caulfied LE, Richard SA, Black RE.

Undernutrition as an underlying cause of malaria morbidity and mortality in children less than five years old.

Am J. Trop Med Hyg. 2004 Aug;71 (2 Suppl): 55-63. Review. PMID: 15331819 (PubMed - indexed for MEDLINE)

Andres E, Loukili NH, Noel E, Kaltenbach G, Abodelgheni MB Perrin AE, Nobler-Dick M, Maloisel F, Schlienger JL, Blickle JF. Vitamin B 12 (cobalamin) deficiency in elderly patients. CMAJ. 2004 Aug 3; 171 (3): 251-9. Review.

Postgrad Med. 2004 Jul; 116 (1) : 57-64

Diabetic retinopathy. Control of systemic factors preserves vision.

Colucciello M.

South Jersey Eye Physicians, Moorestown, New Jersey 80057 USA.

Arch Intern Med. 2004 Jul 12; 164 (13) : 1395-404.

Comment in:

ACP J club. 2005 Jan-Feb; 142 (1) : 8.

Efficacy of pharmacotherapy for weight loss in adults with type 2 diabetes.

Med Clin North Am 2004 Jul;88 94) : 933-45, xi.

Gonadal and erectile dysfunction in diabetes.

Hijazi RA, Betancourt-Albrecht M, Cunningham GR.

Department of Medicine, Veterans Affairs Medical Center, Houston, TX 77030, USA.

Med Clin North Am. 2004 Jul;88 (4) : 911-31, x-xi

Endothelial dysfunction and hypertension in diabetes mellitus.

Dandona P, Chaudhuri A, Aljada A.

Division of Endocrinology, Diabetes, and Metabolism, State University of New York at Buffalo and Kaleida Health, 3 Gates Circle, Buffalo, NY 14209, USA. pdandona@kaleidahealth. org.

Austin, M.A., et al. "Low-Density Lipoprotien Subclass Patterns and Risk of Myocardial Infraction." JAMA 260. (1988): 1917-1921

Baba, T., and S. Neugebauer. "The Link Between Insulin Resistance and Hypertension: Effects of Antihypertesive and Antihyperilipidaemic Drugs on Insulin Sensitivity." Drugs 47 (1994): 383-404.

Pilkis SJ, Granner DK.

Molecular physiology of the regulation of hepatic gluconeogensis.

Annu. Rev. Pysiol; 54: 885-909, 1992

Unger RH, Orci L

Physiology and pathophysiology of glucagons.

R.D. Miller, M.D.

Physiol. Rev. 56: 778-838,1976.

Zimmet PZ, Alberti KGMM.

The changing face of macrovascular disease in non-insulin-dependent diabetes mellitus. An epidemic in progress.

Lancet. 1997;350 (suppl 1) 1-4

Eastman RC, Keen H.

The impact of cardiovascular disease on people with diabetes.

Lancet 1997; 350 (supl 1) 29-32

Des Pres JP, Lamarche B, Mauriege P, et al.

Hyperinsulinemia as an independent risk factor for ischemic heart disease.

N Engl J Med 1996; 334: 952-957

Solymoss BC, Marcil M, Chaour M; et al.

Fasting hyperinsulinism, insulin resistance syndrome, and coronary artery disease in men and women.

Am J Cardio, 1995; 76; 1152-1156.

Koivisto, P. and R.A. Defronzo. "Physical Training and Insulin Sensitivity." Diabetes metabolism Reviews.

Syvanne M, Taskinen MR.

Lipids and lipoproteins as coronary risk factors in non-insulin-dependent diabetes mellitus. Lancet. 1997, 350 (suppl 1) 20-23.

Freund H, Atamian S, Fischer JE.

Chorminm deficiency during total parental nutrition. J Am Heart Assoc. 214: 496-498, 1979.

Anderson RA, Kozlovsky AS.

Chorium intake, absorption and excretion of subjects consuming self selected diets. Am J Clini Nutr 41: 1177-1183, 1985.

Gass M, Dawson-Hughes B. Preventing osteoporosis-related fractures; an overview. Am J Med. 2006 April; 119 (4 Suppl 1); S3-S11. Review. PMID: 16563939 (PubMed-indexed for MEDLINE.

Holick MF.

High prevalence of vitamin D inadequacy and implication for health. Mayo Clini Proc. 2006 Mar; 81 (3) ;353-73. Review. PMID: 16529140 (PubMed—indexed for MEDLINE)

Luba KM, Stulberg DL.

Chronic plaque psoriasis.

Am Fam physician. 2006 Feb;15;73 (4) : 636-44 Review. PMID: 16506705 (Pub—indexed for MEDLINE)

Keusch GT.

What do –omics mean for the science and policy of the nutritional sciences? Am J Clin Nutr. 2006 Feb;83 (2) : 520S-522S. Review PMID: 16470024 (PubMed - indexed for

R.D. Miller, M.D.

MEDLINE)

Penniston KL, Tanumihardjo SA. The acute and chronic toxic effects of vitamin A. Am J Clin Nutr. 2006 Feb; 83 (2) : 191-201. Review. PMID: 16469975 (PubMed—MEDLINE)

Pennisi P, Trombetti A, Rizzoli R.

Glucocorticoid-induced osteoporosis and its treatment. Clin Orthop Relat Res. 2006 Feb; 443-39-47. Review. PMID: 16462424 (PubMed - indexed for MEDLINE)

Am J Clin Nutr. 2004 Dec: 80 (6) : 1492-9

Comment in:

Am J Clin Nuttr. 2004 Dec; 80 (6) : 1492-9

Intakes of whole grains, bran and germ and the risk of coronary heart disease in men. Jensen MK, Koh-Banerjee P, Hu FB, Franz M, Sampson L, Grobaek M, Rimm EB.

J Clin Endocrinal Metab. 2005 Jun; 90 (6) : 3802 author reply 3802

Low-fat high-fiber diet decreased serum and urine androgens in men.

Am J Respir Crit Care Med.. 2004 Aug 1; 170 (3): 279-87 Epub 2004 Apr 29. Dietary fiber and reduced cough with plegm: a cohort study in Singapore.

Butler LM, Koh WP, Lee HP, Yu MC, London SJ.

Dig Dis Sci. 2005 June; 50 (6) : 1107-12

Treatment effects of partially hydrolyzed guar gum on symptoms and quality of life of patients with irritable bowl syndrome. A multicenter randomized open trial.

Parisi G, Bottona E, Carrara M, Cardin F, Faedo A, Goldin D, Mariono M, Pantalena M, Tafner G, Versianelli G, Zilli M, Leandro G.

Paolisso, G., et al. " Pharmacological doses of Vitamin E Improves Insulin Action in Healthy Subjects & Non-Insulin-Dependent Diabetic Patients." American Journal of Nutrition 57. (1993): 650-656.

Reaven, G.M., "Diet and Syndrome X." Current Artherosclerosis Reports 2. (2000): 503-507

J Gerontol A Biol Sci Med Sci 2004 May; 59 (5) : 478-493.

Free radicals: Key to brain aging and heme oxygenase as a cellular response to oxidative stress. Poon HF, Calabrese V. Scapagnini G, Butterfield DA.

Cusin I., et al "Hyperinsulininemia and It's impact on Obesity Resistance." International Journal of Obesity 16. (1992): S1-S11

Farquhaar, J.W., et al. "Glucose, Insulin and Triglycerides Responses toHigh and Low Carbohydrate diets in Man." Journal of Clinical Investigations 45. (1966): 1648-1656

Coulston, A.M., et al. "Persistence of Hypertriglyceridemic Effect of Low Fat High-Carbohydrate Diet in patients with Non-insulin-dependent diabetes mellitus." New England Journal of Medicine 319. (1988): 829-834.

Coulston, A.M., et al. "Persistence of Hypertriglyceridemic Effect of Low-Fat, High-Carbohydrate Diets in NIDDM patients." Diabetes Care 12.. (1989): 94-101.

Ferrannini, E., et al. "Hyperinsulinaemia: The Key Feature of a Cardiovascular and Meabolic Syndrome. Diabetologia 3. (1991): 4116-422

Grag, A., et al. "Comparison of a High-Carbohydrate Diet with a High-Monounsaturated-Fat Diet in Patients with Non-Insulin-Dependent Diabetes Mellitus." New England Journal of Medicine 39 (1988): 824-834.

Flegal, K.M., et al. "Overweight and Obesity in the US: Prevalence and Trends, 1960-1994. International Journal of Obesity 22. (1998): 39-47.

Glass, A.R., "Endoctrine Aspects of Obesity." Medical Clinics of North America 73. (1989): 139-160.

Connolly, J.A., "Obesity increases U.S. health cost by $93 B," Rapid City Journal.

Fontaine, K.R., et al. "Years of Life Due to Obesity." JAMA 289. (2003): 187-193.

Holloszy, J.O., et al. "Effects of Exercise on Glucose Tolerance and Insulin Resistance." Acta Medica Scandinavica 711. (1996): 55-65.

Med Clin North Am. 2004 Jul: 8 (4) : 1037-61, xi-xii

Odeley, F.Q., et al. "Fasting Hyperinsulinemia Is A Predicor of Increased Body Weight Gain and Obesity in Pima Indian Children." diabetes 46. (1997): 1341-1345.

Reaven, G.M., et al. "Role of Insulin in Edogenous Hypertriglycerdemia." Journal of Clinical Investigation 46. (1967): 1756-1767.

Prog Cariovasc Dis. 2006 Jan-Feb; 48 (4) : 270-84. Exercise and the coronary circulation-alterations and adaptations in coronary artery disease. Linke A. Erbs S, Hambrecht R.

J Allergy Clin Immunol. 2006 Feb; 117 (2) : 259-62
Nitric oxide as a clinical guide for asthma management.
Taylor DR.

Crit Care Med. 2005 Dec; 33 (12 Suppl) : 5498-501.
Reactive oxygen species.
Bayir H.

Crit Care Med. 2005 Dec; 33 (12 Suppl) : S492-5.
Nitric oxide: a clinical primer.
Ley RM, Prince JM, Biiliar TR.

Anesth Analg. 2005 Nov; 101 (5) : 1275-87.
Reactive oxygen species as mediators of cardic injury and

R.D. Miller, M.D.

protection: the relevance to anesthesia practice.

Am J Cardiol. 2005 Oct 10; 96 (7B) : 131-241.

Epub 2005 Aug 8.

Understanding nitric oxide physiology in the heart: a nanomedical approach.

Malinski T.

J Clin Invest. 2005 Mar; 115 (3) : 509-17.

NO/redox disequilibrium in the falling heart and cardiovascular system.

Hare JM, Stampler JS.

Crit Care Med. 2005 Mar; 33(3 Suppl) : 5182-7

High frequency oscillatory ventilation and adjunctive therapies: inhaled nitric oxide and prone positioning.

Fan E, Mehta S.

Ischemic heart disease and congest heart failure in diabetic patients.

Wilson Tang WH, Marco A, Young JB.

Department of Cardiovascular Medicine, Cleveland Clinic Foundation

9500 Euclid Avenue, Desk F25, Cleveland, Ohio 44195, USA. tangw@ccf.org

Med Clin North AM. 2004 Jul; 88 (4) : 1001-36, xi

Diabetic nephropathy and retinopathy.

Jawa A, Kcomt J, Fonseca VA.

Section of Endocrinology, Department of Medicine, Tulane University Health Science Center, SL-53, 1430 Tulane Avenue, New Orleans, LA 70112-2699, USA

Med Clin North AM. 2004 Jul;88 (4) : xii

In hospital management of type 2 diabetes mellitus.

Lien LF, Angelyn Bethel M, Feinglos MN. Division of Endocrinology, Metabolism, and Nutrition, Department of Medicine, Duke University Medical, Box 3921, Durham, NC 27710, USA. lien0002@mc.duke.edu

Med Clin North AM 2004 Jul;88 (4) : 1063-84, xii

Acute hyperglycemic crisis in the elderly.

Gaglia JL, Wyckoff J, Abrahamson MJ

Joslin Diabetes Center, Beth Israel Deaconess Medical Center

1 Joslin Place, Boston, MA 02215, USA

Ahmed, M., et al.

"Plasma Glucagons and (-Amino Acid Nitrogen Response to Various Diets in Normal Humans." American Journal of Nutrition33. (1980): 1917-1924

Anderson, J.W. "Fiber and Health: An Overview." American Journal of Gastroenterology 81. (1986)

Insights from calcium and vitamin D.

Am J Clin Nutr. 2003 Nov; 78 (5): 912-9 Review. PMID: 14585642 (PubMed—indexed for MEDLINE)

Wharton B, Bishop N.

Rickets.

Lancet, 2003 Oct 25;362 (9393): 1389-400. Review. PMID: 14585642 (PMID-indexed for MEDLINE)

Congdon NG, Friedmen DS, Lietman T.

Important causes of visual impairment in the world today.

JAMA. 2003 Oct 15;290 (15): 2057-60. Review. No abstract available. PMID: 13559961 (PubMed—indexed for MEDLINE)

Harden CL.

Menopause and bone density issues for women with epilepsy. Neurology. 2003 Sep1;61 (6 Suppl 2):S16-22. Review. PMID: 14504305 (PubMed—indexed for MEDLINE)

Fiechtner JJ.

Hip fracture prevention. Drug therapies and lifestyle and modifications that can reduce risk. Postgrad Med. 2003 Sep; 114 (3): 22-8, 32. Review. PMID: 14503398 (PubMed – indexed for MEDLINE)

Leslie WD, Bernstein CN, Leboff MS.

American Gastroenterology Association Clinical Practice Committee. AGA technical review on osteoporosis in hepatic disorders. Gastroenterology - 2003 Sep; 125 (3) : 941-66. Review. No Abstract available. PMID: 12949738 (PubMed-indexed for MEDLINE)

Pettifor JM.

Nutritional rickets: deficiency of vitamin D, calcium, or both?
Am J Clin Nutr. 2004 Dec; 80 (6 Suppl): 1725S-9S. Review.
PMID: 15585795 (PubMed—indexed for MEDLINE)

Welsh J.

Vitamin D and breast cancer: insights from animal models.
AmJ Clin Nutr. 2004 Dec;80 (6Suppl): 172S-4S. Review.
PMID: 15585794 (PubMed—indexed for MEDLINE)

Cantorna MT, Zhu Y, Froicu M, Wittke A.

Vitamin D status, 1.25-dihydroxyvitamin D3, and the immune
system.

Am J Clin Nutr. 2004 Dec; 80 (6Suppl): 1717S-20S. Review.
PMID: 15585793 (PubMed-index for MEDLINE)

Calvo MS, Whiting SJ, Barton CN. Vitamin D fortification in
the United State and Canada: current status and data needs.

Am J Clin Nutr. 2004 Dec;80 (6 Suppl): 1710S-6S,Review.
PMID: 15585792 (PubMed - indexed for MEDLINE)

Weisberg P, Scanlon KS, Li R, Cogswell ME. Nutritional
rickets amoung children in the United States review of cases
reported between 1986 and 2003.

Am J Clin Nutr. 2004 Dec; 80 (6 Suppl): 1697S-705S. Review.
PMID: 13585790 (PubMed—indexed for MEDLINE)

DeLuca HF.

Overview of general physiologic features and functions of
vitamin D.

Am J Clin Nutr. 2004 Dec; 80 (6Suppl): 1689S-96S. Review.
PMID: 15585789 (PubMed—indexed for MEDLINE)

Bray, G., B. York, J Delaney.

A survey of the opinions of obesity experts on the cause and treatment of obesity.

Am J of Clin Nutr 55 1992: 151-154S

Blundell, J

Serotonnin and the biology of feeding. Am J Clin Nutr 55; 1992:155S

Degraffin C, Hulshof, Westrate JA, P Jas.

Short-term effects of different amounts of protein, fat and carbohydrates on satiety.

Am J Clin Nutr 55; 1992: 33-38

Jenkins D, JA, et al

Nibbling versus gorging: Metabolic advantages of increased meal frequency. N Eng j Med 321;1989

Brand Miller, J.

The importance of glyemic index diabetes.

Am J Clin Nutr 59 (suppl.) 194: 747 S-752S.

UUsitupa M.

Fructose in the diabetic diet.

Am J Clin Nutr. 59 (supl.)1994: 753 S.

Foster-Powell K, Miller JB

International tables of glycemic index.

Am J Clin Nutr 62, 1995

Jenkins DJA, Wolever TMS, Taloe RH, et al.

Glycemic index of foods:

A physiological basis for carbohydrates exchange.

For indicating need for weight management.

Brit Med J 311; 1995 158 - 161

Kuczmarski Rj, et al.

Increasing prevalence of overweigh among US adults.

The National Health and Nutrition examination surveys, 1960-1991. J of the Am Med Assoc. 272, 1994: 205-211

B-Vitamin Treatment Trialists' Collaboration.

Homocysteine-lowering trials for prevention of cardiovascular events: a review of the design and power of the large randomized trials.

Am Heart J. 2006 Feb; 151 (2) : 282-7. Review. PMID: 16442889 (PUBMED—indexed for MEDLINE)

Kripke C.

Is oral vitamin B12 as effective as intramuscular injection? Am Fam Physician. 2006 Jan 11; 73 (10 :65). Review. No abstract available.

PMID: 16417065 (PubMed—indexed for MEDLINE)

(No authors listed)

R.D. Miller, M.D.

Vitamin supplements.

Obstet Gynecol. 2006 Jan: 107 (1) : 174-6. Review. No abstract available.

PMID: 16394056 (PubMed– indexed for MEDLINE)

Garland CF, Garland FC, Gorham ED, Lipkin M,

Newmark H, Mohr SB, Holick MF.

The role of vitamin D in cancer prevention.

Am J Public Health. 2006 Feb; 96 (2) : 252-61

Epub 2005 Dec 27. Review. PMID: 16322775 (PubMed– indexed for MEDLINE)

Raisz LG,

Pathogenesis of osteoporosis: concepts, conflicts, and prospects.

J Clin Invest. 2005 Dec: 115 (12) :3318-25 Review. PMID: 16322775 (PubMed– indexed for MEDLINE)

Kannus P, Sievanen H, Palvaned M, Jarvinen T, Parkkari J.

Prevention of falls and consequent injuries in elderly people.

Lancet. 2005 Nov 26; 366 (9500) : 1885-93. Review. PMID: 16310556 (PubMed –indexed for MEDLINE)

Collier, G.R. et al. "Low Glycemic Index Starchy Foods Improve Glucose Control and Lower Serum Cholesterol in Diabetic Children."

Diabetes Nutr Metabolism 1. (1988):11-19.

Frost G., "Dietary Advise Based on the Glycemic Index Improves Dietary Profile and Metabolic control in type 2 diabetic patients." Diabetic Medicine 11. (1993): 397-401.

Griendling, K.K., et al. "Oxidative Stress and Cardiovascular Disease." Circulation 96. (1997): 3264-3265.

Hu, F. et al. "Dietary Fat intake and the Risk of Coronary Heart Disease in Women." New England Journal of Medicine 337, (1997) 1491-1499.

Haber, G.B. et al. "Depletion and Disruption of dietary Fiber: Effect on Satiety, Plasma-Glucose , and serum Insulin." Lancet 2. (1977): 679-682.

Hu, F., et al "Trends in the Incidence of Coronary Heart Disease and changes in diet and Lifestyle in Women." New England Journal of Medicine. 343, (2000): 530-537.

Grundy, S.M. "Comparison of Monosaturated fatty Acids and Carbohydrates for lowering plasma Cholesterol." New England Journal of Medicine 314. (1986) 745-748.

Foster, D. "Insulin Resistance-A Secret Killer?" New England Journal of Medicine 320. (1989): 733-734.

Foster-Powell, K. and J.B. Miller. "International Tables of Glycemic Index." American Journal of Clinical Nutrition 62. (1995): 871-890S

Halliwell, B., and J. Gutteridge. "The Antioxidants of Human Extra Cellular Fluids." Archives of biochemistry and

R.D. Miller, M.D.

Biophysiology 280. (1990):1-8

Jenkins, D., et al "Glycemic Index of Foods: A physiological Basis for Carbohydrate Exchange." American Reaven, GM et al "Relationship Between Glucose Toleranc Insulin Secretion, and Insulin Action of Non-Obese Individuals with varying degrees of glucose Tolerance." Diebetologia 32. (1989): 52-55.

Nuttall, F.Q., et al. "Effects of Protein Ingestion on the Glucose and Insulin response to a Standardize Oral glucose load." Diabetes Care 7. (1984): 465-470.

Reaven, G.M,et al. "Insulin Resistance and Hyperinsulinemia in Individuals with Small, Dense, Low Density Lipoprotein Particles." Journal of Clinical Investigation 92.(1998): 141-146.

Rasmussen, O.W., et al. "Effects on blood Pressure, Glucose, and Lipid Levels of a High– Carbohydrate Diet in Non-Insulin dependent subjects." Diabetes Care 16. (1993): 37-46.

Reaven, G.M., et al. Insulin Resistance and Hyperinsulinemia in Individuals with Small, Dense, Low Density Lipoprotein Particles." Journal of Clinical Investigation 92. (1998) 142-146.

Reaven, G.M., Y. Chen. "Role of Insulin in Regulation of Lipoprotein Metabolism in Diabetes." Diabetes/Metabolism Rev. 4. (1998): 639-652.

Reaven, G.M., "Banting Lecture 1988: Role of Insulin Resistance in Human Disease." Diabetes 37 (1989): 1595-1607.

Stamler, J., et al. "Prevention and Control of Hypertension by Nutritional-Hygienic Means. "Journal of the American Medical Association243. (1980): 1819-1823.

Rosman, P., et al. "Regulation of Glucagon Release from Pancreatic A-Cells." Biochemical Pharmacology 41. (1991): 1783-1790.

Liu, S., et al. "A Prospective Study of Dietary Glycemic Load, Carbohydrate Intake and Risk of coronary Artery Disease in US Women." American Journal of Clinical Nutrition 71. (2000): 1455-1461.

Miller, J.B., "The Glycemic Index is Easy and works in practice." diabetes Care 20. (1997): 1628-1629.

Libman, I., and S.A. Arlanian. "Type 2 Diabetes Mellitus: No Longer Just Adults." Pediatrics Annals 28. (1999): 589-593.

Meyer, J.B., et al. "Carbohydrates, Dietary Fiber and Incidents type 2 Diabetes in Older women. American Journal of Clinical Nutrition 71. (2000): 921-930.

Levine, G.N., et al. " Ascorbic Acid Reverses Endothelial Vasomotor Dysfunction in Patients with Coronary Artery Disease." Circulation 93. (1996): 1107-1113.

Metges, C.C. and C.A., Barth. "Metabolic Consequences of a High Dietary-Protein Intake in Adulthood: Assessment of the Available Evidence." Journal of Nutrition 130. (2000): 886-

R.D. Miller, M.D.

889.

Leon, A.S., et al. "Effects of Vigorous Walking Program on Body composition, and Cardiovascular and Lipid Metabolism of Obese Young Men." Journal of Clinical Nutrition 33 (1979): 1776-1787.

McNamara, D., "Regular Breakfast Eaters at Lower Risk for Obesity." Family Practice News 15. 15 Many 2003.

Manson, J., and S. Bassuk. "Obesity in the United States: a Fresh Look at It's High Toll." JAMA 289. (2003): 229-230.

Mayer-Davis, E.J., et al. "Intensity and Amount of Physical Activity in Relation to Insulin Sensitivity." JAMA 279. (1998): 669-674.

Reaven, G.M., "Syndrome X: 6 Years Later." Journal of Internal Medicine Suppl 736. (1994): 13-22.

Manson JE, et al.
Body Weight Mortality Amount Women.
N Eng J Med 333; 1995:205-211.

Reaven GM.
Role of Insulin Resistance in Human Disease.
Diabetes, 1988; 37: 1595-1607.

Campbell PJ, Gerick JE

Impact of obesity action in volunteers with normal glucose tolerance: Demonstration of a threshold for adverse effect of obesity.

J Clin endocrinology and Metabolism 70, 1114-1118, 1990

Perriello G, Miscericordis P, Volpi E,

Pampanelli S, Santensanio F, Burnette P, Bolli GB

Contributions of obesity to insulin to resistance in non-insulin dependent diabetes mellitus.

J Clin Endocrinology and Metabolism 80 (8): 2464-9- Aug, 1995

Mayer-Davis ED' Agostino R Karter AJ, Haffer SM, Rewers MJ, Saad M, Bergman RN. Instensity and amount of physical activity. The insulin resistance atherosclerosis study. JAMA 279: 669-674, 1998.

Nolan JJ, Judvik B, Beerdsen P, Joyce M, Olefsky J.

Improvement in glucose tolerance and insulin resistance in obsess subjects treated with troglitazone.

N Eng J. Med 3;331 (18) 1188-93, 1994 Nov.

Witztum JL, Steinberg D.

Disorders of lipid metabolism—the hyperlipoptienemeans.

Decil's Textbook Med. 1086-1087. 1987.

Goldfine IG

The insulin receptor molecular biology and transmembrane signaling. Endor. Rev 8:235-255. 1987.

R.D. Miller, M.D.

Holloszy, J.O., et al. "Effects of Exercise on Glucose Tolerance and Insulin Resistance." Acta Medica Scandinavica 711. (1992): 129-141.

Boosalis MG, Evans GW, McLain CJ.

Impaired handling of orally administration zinc in pancreatic insufficiency.

Am J Clini Nutr 46:511-517.

Krieger I, Statter M.

Tryophan Defiance and picolinate:

Effect on zinc metabolism and clinical manifestion of pellagra.

Am J Clini Nutr 46: 511-517.

Schroeder HA.

The role of chromium in mammalian nutrition.

Am J Nutr 21: 230-244, 1968.

Jeejeebhoy JN, Chu RC, Marliss EB,

Greenberg R, Bruce-Robertson AS.

Chromiun deficiency, glucose intolerance and neupropathy reversed in a patient receiving long-term total parental nutrition.

Am J Clin Nutr 30:531-538, 1977.

Orish JR, Brown s, Scherwitz LW and others.

Can lifestyle changes reverse coronary heart disease?

Lancet 366, 1990.

Crouse Jr.

Gender, lipoproteins, diet and cardiovascular risk. Lancet 1:318, 1989.

Brunzell JD, Austin MA

Plasma triglyceride levels and coronary heart disease.

N Eng J Med. 320:1273, 1989.

Paffenbarger RS, Hale WE.

Work activity and coronary heart mortality.

N Eng J Med 292:545, 1975.

Anderson JW, Johnstone BM, Cook-Newell ME.

Metalanalysis of the effects of soy protein intake on serum lipids.

E Eng Med 333: 276-282, 1995.

Jenkins, D., et al. "Glycemic Index of Foods: A Physiological Basis for Carbohydrate Exchange." American Journal of Clinical Nutrition 34. (1981): 362-366.

McKeever TM, Britton J.

Diet and Asthma.

Am J Respir Crit Care Med. 2004 Oct 1: 170 (7): 725-9.

PMID: 15256393 (PubMed—indexed for MEDLINE).

Gasche C, Lomer MC, Cavill I, Weiss G.

R.D. Miller, M.D.

Iron, anaemi, and inflammatory bowel diseases.

Gut. 2004 Aug; 53 (8): 1190-7. Review.

PMID: 15247190 (PubMed—indexed for MEDLINE).

Splaver A, Lamas GA, Hennekens CH.

Homocysteline and cardiovascular disease: biological mechanism, obersvational epidemiology, and the need for randomized trials.

Am Heart J. 2004 Jul; 148 (1): 34-40. Review. PMID: 15215789 (PumMed—indexed for MEDLINE)

Moorman PG, Terry PD.

Consumption of diary products and the risk of breast cancer: a review of the literature.

Am J Clin Nutr. 2004 Jul; 80 (1): 5-14. Review.

PMID: 15213021 (PubMed - indexed for MEDLINE)

Gazadar AF, Miyajima K, Reddy J, Sathyanarayana UG, Shigematsu H, Suzuki M, Takahashi T, Shivapurkar N. Molecular targets for cancer therapy and prevention. Chest. 2004 May; 125 (5 Suppl): 97S-101S. Review PMID: 15136434 (PubMed-indexed for MEDLINE)

Zemel MB.

Role of calcium and dairy products in energy partitioning and weight management.

Am J Clin Nutr. 2004 May; 79 (5): 907S-912S. Review. PMID: 15113738 (PubMed - indexed for MEDLINE)

Hollis BW, Wagner CL.

Assessment of dietary vitamin D requirements during pregnancy and lactation.

Am J Clin Nutr. 2004 May: 79 (79) 717-26. Review. PMID: 15113709 (PubMed - indexed for MEDLINE)

Bilezikian JP, Silvergerg SJ.

Clinical practice. Asymptomatic primary hyperparathyroidism.

N Engl J Med. 2004 Apr 22; 350 (17): 1746-51.

Review. No abstract available.

PMID: 15103001 (PubMed - indexed for MEDLINE)

Inzucchi SE.

Understanding hypercalcemia. Its metabolic basis, signs, and symptoms.

Postgrad Med. 2004 Apr; 115 (4) 69-70, 73-6. Review. PMID: 15005538 (PubMed - indexed for MEDLINE)

Qureshi A, Lee-Choing T Jr.

Medications and their effects on sleep.

Med Clin North Am. 2004 May:88 (3): 751-66, x.

Review. No abstract available. PMID: 15087214 (PubMed - indexed for MEDLINE)

Reid KJ, Chang AM, Zee PC.

Circadian rhythm sleep disorders.

Med Clin North Am. 2004 May; 88 (3): 631-51, viii. Review. No abstract available. PMID: 15087208 (PubMed - indexed for MEDLINE)

Pawley N. Bishop NJ.

Prenatal and infant predictors of bone health: the influence of vitamin D.

Am J Clin Nutr. 2004 Dec; 80 (6 Suppl): 1748S–51S. Review. PMID: 15585799 (PubMed - indexed for MEDLINE)

Specker B.

Vitamin D requirements during pregnancy.

Am J Clin Nutr. 2004 Dec; 80 (6 Suppl) : 1740S-7S. Review. PMID: 15585798 (PubMed - indexed for MEDLINE)

Weaver CM, Fleet JC.

Vitamin D requirements: current and future.

Am J clin Nutr. 2004 Dec; 80 (6Suppl): 1725S-9S. Review. Erratum in: Am J Clin Nutr. 2005 Mar; 81 (3): 729. PMID: 15585797 (PubMed - indexed for MEDLINE)

Fleet JC.

Genomic and proteomic approaches for probing the role of vitamin D in health.

Am J Clin Nutr. 2004 Dec; 80 (6 Suppl): 1730S-4S. Review. PMID: 15585796 (PubMed - indexed for MEDLINE)

Wang L, Levin MS.

Suppression of FGF signaling: a putative mechanism for the chemo preventive effects of acyclic retinoid inn hepatocellular carcinoma.

Gastroenterology. 2005 Jan; 128 (1): 228-31. Review. No abstract available. PMID: 15633140 (PubMed - indexed for

MEDLINE)

Maalouf NM, Shane E.

Osteoporosis after solid organ transplantation.

J Clin Endocrinal Metab. 2005 Apr;90 (4): 2456-65. Epub 2004 Dec 28. Review. Erratum in: J Clin Endocrinal Metab. 2005 Jul; 90 (7): 4118. PMID: 15623822 PubMed - indexed for MEDLINE)

Postgrad Med. 2005 Nov; 118 (5): 19-26, 29

Treatment of diabetes in the elderly. Addressing its complexities in this high-risk group.

Sakharova OV, Inzucchi SE.

Section of Endocrinology, Yale University School of Medicine, New Haven, Connecticut 06520, USA

J Fam Pract. 2005 Oct: Suppl: S1-8

The role of basal insulin in type 2 diabetes management.

Brunton Sa, white JR Jr, Renda SM

Arch Phys Med Rehabil. 2004 Jul;

85 (7 Suppl3) : S76-82; quiz S83-4,

Selected medical management of the older rehabilitative patient.

Lin JL, Armour D.

Department of Internal Medicine, Emory University School of Medicine, Atlanta, GA, USA

John.Lin@med.va.gov

Bjorke Monsen AL, Ueland PM.

Hemocysteine and methlmallonic acid in diagnosis and risk assessment from infancy to adolescence.

Am J Clin Nutr. 2003 Jul; 78 (1) : 7-21. Review

PMID: 12816766 (PubMed indexed for MEDLINE)

Antony AC.

Vegetarianism and vitamin B-12 (cobalamin) deficiency.

Am J Clin Nutr. 2003 Jul; 78 (1) :3-6. Review. No abstract available.

PMID: 12816765 (PubMed indexed for MEDLINE)

Powers HJ.

Riboflavin (vitamin B-2) and health.

Am J clin Nutr. 2003 Jun; 77 (6) : 1352-60. Review. PMID: 12716711 (PubMed - indexed for MEDLINE)

Mactier H, Weaver LT.

Vitamin A and preterm infants: what we know, what we don't know, and what we need to know. Arch Dis Child Fetal Neonatal Ed. 2005 Mar; 90 (2); F103-8. Review. PMID: 15724031 (PubMed - indexed for MEDLINE)

Grimes PE.

New insights and new therapies in vitiligo. JAMA. 2005 Feb 9; 293 (6): 730-5. Review. No abstract available.

PMID: 15701915 (PubMed - indexed for MEDLINE)

Lyman D.

Undiagnosed vitamin D deficiency in the hospitalized patient. AM Fam Physician. 2005 Jan 156: 71 (2): 299-304. Review. PMID: 15686300 (PubMed - indexed for MEDLINE)

Mignini LE, Latthe PM, Villar J, Kilby MD, Carroli G, Khan KS. Mapping the theories of preeclampsia: the role of homocysteine. Obstet Gynocol. 2005 Feb; 105 (2): 411-25. Review. PMID: 15684173 (PubMed—indexed for MEDLINE)

Carroll MF, Schade DS.

A practical approach to hyercalcemia.

Am Fam Physician. 2003 May 1; 67 (9): 1959-66 Review. PMID: 12751658 (PubMed - indexed for MEDLINE)

Singh J, Moghal N, Pearce SH, Cheetham T.

The investigation of hypocalcaemia and rickets. Arch Dis Child. 2003 May;88 (5) : 403-7. Review. PMID: 12716711 (PubMed—indexed for MEDLINE)

Hollick MF.

Vitamin D: importance in the prevention of cancers, type I diabetes, heart disease, and osteoporosis. Am J Clin Nutr: 2004 Mar; 79 (3): 362-71

Review. Erratum in: Am J Clin Nutr. 2004 May; 79 (5): 890. PMID: 14985208 (PubMed—indexed for MEDLINE)

Barnes TC, Bucknall RC.

Vitamin D deficiency in a patient with systemic lupus erythematosus.

Rheumatology)Oxford). 2004 Mar; 43 (3): 393-4. Review. No abstract available. PMID: 14963211 (PubMed - indexed for MEDLINE)

Harris RJ.

Nutrition in the 21st century: what is going wrong.

Arch Dis Child. 2004 Feb;89 (2): 154-8. Review.

PMID: 14736634 (PubMed—indexed for MEDLINE)

Kristal AR.

Vitamin A. retinoids and carotenoids as chemo preventive agents for prostate cancer.

J Urol. 2004 Feb; 171 (2Pt 2): S54-8; discussion S58.

Review.

PMID: 14713755 (PubMed - indexed for MEDLINE)

Price DK, Franks ME, Figg WD.

Genetic variations in the vitamin D receptor, androgen receptor and enzymes that regulate androgen metabolism.

J Urol. 2004 Feb; 171 (2 Pt2): S45-9; discussion S49.

Review.

PMID: 14713753 (PubMed - indexed for MEDLINE)

Heaney RP.

Vitamin D. nutritional deficiency, and the medical paradigm.

J Clin Endocrinal Metab. 2003 Nov;88 (11): 5107-8

Review. No abstract available.

PMID: 14602734 (PubMed—indexed for MEDLINE)

Sanz MA, Tailman MS, Lo-Coco F.

Tricks of the trade for the appropriate management of newly diagnosed acute promelyocytic leukemia.

Blood. 2005 Apr 15' 105 (8): 3019-25. Equb 2004 Dec 16.

Review.

PMID: 15604216 (PubMed—indexed for MEDLINE)

Dawson-Hughes B.

Racial/ethnic considerations in making recommendations for vitamin D for adult and elderly men and women.

Am J clin Nutr. 2004 Dec; 80 (6 Suppl): 1763S-6S. Review.
PMID: 15585802 (PubMed—indexed for MEDLINE)

Greer FR.

Issues in establishing vitamin D recommendations for infants and children.

Am J Clin Nutr. 2004 Dec; 80 (6 Supl): 17559S-62S.

Review.

PMID: 15585801 (PubMed - indexed for MEDLINE)

Kelly BF, Burroughs M, Mertens M.

Clinical inquiries. Dous treatment of acne with Retin A and tetracycline cause adverse effects?

J Fam Pract. 2004 Apri; 53 (4): 316-8.

Review. No abstract available.

PMID: 15068778 (PubMed - indexed for MEDLINE)

Demay M.

R.D. Miller, M.D.

Muscle: a nontraditional 1, 25-dihydroxyvitamin D target tissue exhibiting classic hormone-dependent vitamin D receptor actions.

Endocrinology. 2003 Dec; 144 (12): 5135-7. Review.

No abstract available.

PMID: 14645209 (PubMed - indexed for MEDLINE)

Stephen, A.M., et al. "intake of Carbohydrate and Its Components - International Comparisons, Trends Overtime, and Effects of Changing to Low-Fat Diets." American Journal of Clinical Nutrition 62. (1995):851S-867S.

Ross, R., "Atherosclerosis—an Inflammoatory Diseas." New England Journal of Medicine 340. (1999): 115-123.

Salmeron, J., et al. "Dietary Fiber, Glycemic Load and Risk of on-Insulin Dependent Diabetes Mellitus in Women." JAMA 277. (1997): 472-477.

Skov, A.R., et al. "Randomized Trial on Protei vs Carbohydrate in Ad Libitum Fat Reduced Diet for the Treatment of Obesity." International Journal of Obesity 23. (1999): 451-458.

Schlosser, Eric. Fast Food Nation. Mifflin Company, (2002)

Wolever, T., et al. "Beneficial Effect of Low Glycemic Index Diet in Type 2 Diabetes." Diabetic Medicine 9. (1992): 451-458.

Woolf AD, Akesson K.

Preventing fractures in elderly people.

BMJU, 203 Jul 12; 327 (7406): 89-95.

Review. No abstract available.

Erratum in BMJ 2003 Sep 20; 327 (7416): 663.

PMID: 12855529 (PubMed - indexed for MEDLINE)

Bischoff—Ferrari HA, Dawson-Hughes, Willet WC,

Staehelin HB, Bazemore MG, Zee RY, Wong JB.

Effect of Vitamin D on falls: a meta-analysis.

JAMA. 2004 Apr 28; 291 (16): 1999-2006. Review. PMID: 15113819 (PubMed - indexed for MEDLINE)

TESTIMONIALS

"I not only like your plan, I like you too!"

Mary Beth T.

"I love bread, potatoes and sweets and that's all I've been eating and feel so crappy, can you help me?" "Sure I can, Nurse bring me the whip! When someone is that honest they can definitely be helped and I tell them they are my new challenge."

Dr. Miller

"When I go to restaurants people think I'm looking around at all the beauty there, but I'm seeing if Dr.Miller is in the room before I order."

Sarah P.

"I'm eating more protein at every meal where I can; I lose 7-10 pounds every month."

Wendy S.

"All truckers need to read your book doc - I will loan mine out regularly."

Mac H.

"I'm going on a cruise so don't be mad when I get back cause I usually gain about eight pounds." "Not this time, it will not only be fun, but you'll lose weight, so sit down, relax and learn how." At the next visit she had a big smile and lost seven pounds, and said, "Your right it was easy."

Elizabeth C.

"I have been frustrated for years and a few simple things were all I needed. Thanks Doc."

Carol N.

"You make it sound easy, but it's not. Breaking old habits takes grit!"

Judy H.

"Doctor, do you ever slip? I sure do, when traveling and someone hands me a crusty apricot fried pie. Nobody is perfect. When you fall off the track just get right back on."

Dr. Miller

"I tried everything and couldn't lose an ounce now I lose ounces."

Virgina S.

"Both my parents are obese with diabetes and blood pressure problems and I see now I don't have to be also. Thanks!"

Paul J.

"I've stopped trying to do so many things and do what you say and the weight is coming off."

Linda H.